THE
Fibromyalgia
RELIEF BOOK

Also by Miryam Ehrlich Williamson

Fibromyalgia: A Comprehensive Approach

THE
Fibromyalgia
RELIEF BOOK

---

213 IDEAS FOR IMPROVING
YOUR QUALITY OF LIFE

Miryam Ehrlich Williamson

FOREWORD BY MARY ANNE SAATHOFF, R.N., B.S.N.

WALKER AND COMPANY   NEW YORK

First published in the United States of America in 1998 by
Walker Publishing Company, Inc.

Published simultaneously in Canada by Thomas Allen & Son Canada, Limited, Markham, Ontario

Library of Congress Cataloging-in-Publication Data
Williamson, Miryam Ehrlich.
The Fibromyalgia relief book: 213 ideas for improving your quality of life / Miryam Ehrlich Williamson; foreword by Mary Anne Saathoff.
p.   cm.
Includes bibliographical references and index.
ISBN 0-8027-7553-5 (pbk.)
1. Fibromyalgia—Popular works.   I. Title.
RC927.3.W534   1998
616.7'4—DC21   98-15697
CIP

Book design by M. J. DiMassi

Printed in the United States of America

2   4   6   8   10   9   7   5   3   1

*In memory of Virginia Bullard Glennon
(February 11, 1933–February 3, 1998),
my soul sister, whose wisdom informs this book
and who taught me, in her last months, never
to be too busy for the important things.*

CONTENTS

Foreword   *Mary Anne Saathoff, R.N., B.S.N.*   xi
Acknowledgments   xv

INTRODUCTION: FIBROMYALGIA AND THE QUALITY OF
    YOUR LIFE   1

1. TAKE THE PAIN OUT OF HOUSEHOLD ACTIVITIES   10
       Cleaning   11
       Cooking and After-Meal Cleanup   16
       Shopping for Food   20
       Laundry and Sewing   21
       Home Modifications   23

2. MAXIMIZE MOMENTS OF PLEASURE   24
       Gardening   24
       Entertaining   27
       The Holidays Need Not Be a Pain   29

3. STRATEGIES AT WORK   33
       Accommodations on the Job   33
       Sitting for Your Living   40
       Repetitive Strain Injury   42
       Working Out at Work   52

4. GOING PLACES WITH FIBROMYALGIA   55
       Airports and Airplanes   56
       Time Zone Changes and Jet Lag   59

Contents

Traveling by Car   61
Visiting   65
Walking   68

5. To Sleep, Perchance to Dream   73
   Sleep Disrupters   75
   Preparations That Promote Sleep   78
   Sleep Hygiene   82
   Don't Just Lie There   86
   Wakening Too Often or Too Early   88

6. Committed Relationships   91
   Emotional Strains   91
   Sexual Intimacy   95
   Dialogue   98
   Meeting Each Other's Needs   101

7. Mind and Body   106
   Mental Responses to Pain   107
   Mood and Stress   110
   Cognitive Problems   119
   Energy Conservation   124

8. Fight Back with Good Nutrition   127
   You Are What You Eat   129
   Vitamin Supplements   131
   Mineral Supplements   135
   Amino Acids   136
   Yeast Overgrowth: Is There a Connection?   140
   Your Responsibilities and Risks   143

9. Exercise to Combat Depression and Pain   145
   The Benefits of Exercise   147
   The Role of Posture in Musculoskeletal Pain   154

10. Standing Up for Yourself   157
    Learn Everything You Can   157

Build Your Support System   159
Assemble Your Medical Team   160
Try Various Approaches   170
Raise Fibromyalgia Awareness in Your Community   174

Resources   177
Notes   195
Index   197

The fibromyalgia syndrome is a condition of musculoskeletal pain and severe fatigue accompanied by disturbed, nonrestorative sleep. An assortment of other symptoms can and often do accompany these three principal manifestations of fibromyalgia. More women than men are affected, and it can develop in people of all ages, including children. Far from being a rare condition, it occurs in at least 2 percent of the adult population in the United States. The possibility of developing fibromyalgia also increases as one ages, with over 7 percent of women between the ages of sixty and seventy-nine having this condition. Although much research is being done, neither the cause of nor the cure for this condition has yet been discovered.

A diagnosis of fibromyalgia may be made quickly by a physician who understands this disorder, but it may be overlooked for far too long by one who does not. As yet, there are no laboratory tests or procedures that prove fibromyalgia's existence. Diagnosis is based on the history of symptoms, accompanied by a brief physical examination in which the physician palpates various areas of the body called tender points. Although there are many possible tender points, only eighteen of the most common ones are usually checked. Pain upon pressure on eleven of these areas confirms the diagnosis.

Almost always, people experience a great sense of relief when a name is given to symptoms that have seemed mysterious and frightening. You may initially be glad to hear that your physician doesn't consider fibromyalgia to be a serious disorder. Physicians say this because, by their standards, a "serious" condition is one that will damage vital organs of the body or even kill those who suffer from it. Fibromyalgia does not lead to either of these outcomes. However, you may soon disagree with this evaluation because fibromyalgia can, indeed, have a serious impact on you. Many people will find their lives have changed in ways they do not appreciate or enjoy.

Treatments offered by the physician are very helpful for some people. Prescriptions for muscle-relaxing medications and pills that can help relieve disturbed sleep can make a real difference. However, not everyone experiences relief with medications, and there may be bothersome or intolerable side effects. The recommendation to start an aerobic exercise program, which is one of the most effective fibromyalgia treatments identified to date, may prove difficult for some to implement and impossible for others.

If you experience continued pain, fatigue, and sleep difficulties after diagnosis, you may visit other doctors, hoping for a quick solution. You may be disappointed that there are not yet any easy answers. You might strive ever harder to make the disagreeable aspects of fibromyalgia disappear, but this does not work and leads only to increased stress and escalating pressures. You may grieve for your past life, deny the reality of the present, and experience anger and depression.

Not everyone will go through this difficult time following their fibromyalgia diagnosis. Some people are affected only mildly. Others may go through these stages to a lesser degree but are able to find ways to manage effectively. Many people, however, will need to do some serious thinking in order to discover how to live with this "not serious" condition that is substantially affecting their quality of life.

Often the first significant advance is made when you decide that you will take charge of your own life. You realize that it is up to you to determine whether you're going to feel worse or whether you're going to feel better. This is a critical decision. It will take you from the passive role of victim and place you in a position of strength from which you can now choose how to proceed. Although your doctor can help, what you are able to do for yourself will be every bit as important, if not more so.

The fact that you have chosen to read this book is a sign that you intend to take control of your life with fibromyalgia. Educate yourself and learn everything you can about this condition, because this knowledge will increase your strength. You will understand that trying ever harder is not the answer but trying "smarter" can be. Investigate the many and varied approaches that have been helpful to others and see if they work for you. If necessary, consider some changes in your lifestyle— not because you have to but because you choose to improve the quality of your life by doing so. Sooner or later, something *will* make a difference.

Reach out to others with fibromyalgia by reading their own stories or meeting and talking with them. Not only is there much to be learned from them, but there is great comfort in coming together and helping each other. You will feel a strong bond with others who know how you feel and who are eager to share their experiences. It can even be possible to laugh about some of your symptoms, which is an excellent pain reliever all by itself.

By taking control of your life, you will learn techniques and skills that will be helpful not just in managing your fibromyalgia but in every other aspect of your life. This strategy is not easy, but the rewards are priceless. Don't be impatient about improving—there need not be deadlines, as you are always a "work in progress." You have empowered yourself and can face the future with strength and hope, knowing that it *is* possible to live well and enjoyably, even with fibromyalgia.

Mary Ann Saathoff, R.N., B.S.N.
President, Fibromyalgia Alliance of America
Columbus, Ohio

ACKNOWLEDGMENTS

The experiences, concerns, and ideas of hundreds of people went into the making of this book. I am grateful to all of them for sharing a part of their lives with me. Special thanks go to Sue Ellen Adkins, Anita Almond, Cyndi Ask, Richard Ask, Michael Baugh, Carolyn Blake, Ann Bradley, Fiona Brown, Carolynne Butters, Tracey Ann Carruthers, Anne-Marie Clanton, Juliana Crouch, Barbara Dawkins, Sherry DiStefano, Cheryl A. Doan, Chris Ford, Marcia Frost, Saundra Gaines, Gillian Gardner, Eileen Glaser, Ted Glaser, Betsy Jacobson, Karen Largent, Shauna Lee Manning, Suzanne Lerner, Donna M. Lindsay, Greg Lovecamp, Janine Lovecamp, Christopher Lord, James Oppenheimer, Penelope Owen, Beverly Kay Phillips, Jack Rector, Sheri Rector, Mary Anne Saathoff, B.S., R.N., Ann Sciabarrasi, O.T.R., Rita Shaw, Jim Sheetz, Helen Shortland, Joyce Summers, Robert Summers, Gordon Thomas, Lori Sova Tillson, Anna Ulshafer, Margaret Unruh, Christine Vanditelli, Jane Walpole, Susan Milstrey Wells, and Eddie Whidden.

No writer could hope for a more patient and thorough editor than Jacqueline Johnson, nor a more supportive agent than Nina Ryan. And to my husband and best friend, Ed Hawes, go great gobs of gooey gratitude for absorbing much of the stress that goes along with the writing of a book, and for bringing joy to my life.

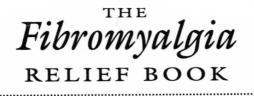

THE
Fibromyalgia
RELIEF BOOK

Introduction

Fibromyalgia and the Quality of Your Life

Imagine this: You have come to live in a new place where the rules are different from those you are accustomed to. You didn't come here of your own free will, but there's every reason to believe this is where you're going to live for the rest of your life. You have two choices: You can complain about the bad luck that brought you here, or you can fight back against that luck, finding ways to make your life here as rich and full and enjoyable as possible. Which do you choose?

Fibromyalgia (FM) is that place. We who inhabit it must adapt to its lifestyle to live well and in reasonable comfort. Understanding as much as I can about fibromyalgia and its symptoms has given me a sense of control over my daily life that brightens my outlook and makes my days manageable—and often even pleasant. I have learned about the contributions that good nutrition and physical activity make to my well-being. I've discovered techniques that get me to sleep and help me wake rested and ready to start the day. I have found ways to reduce the kinds of stress that come from pain, difficult relationships, and my own unrealistically high standards.

I acquired this understanding while researching and writing *Fibromyalgia: A Comprehensive Approach*, the book *I* needed to find when *I* was diagnosed. It didn't exist, so I wrote it. Writing the book brought me into contact with some of fibromyalgia's foremost medical researchers and with hundreds of fellow sufferers on the Internet and in several different support groups. After the book was published I met even more people involved in the research and treatment of fibromyalgia at conferences, where sometimes I listened and sometimes I spoke. By now, I have addressed more than a dozen support groups across the United States. Each time, I have met people with fibromyalgia who have shared with me their unique experiences, thoughts, and feelings. These days I spend about half my time as a peer counselor in one-to-one conversations on the telephone, on the Internet, and in person, offering emotional support, encouragement, and information to people determined to control their own lives the way I do mine. We learn from each other. My life is richer as a result of these conversations.

In 1993, when I got my fibromyalgia diagnosis, I was barely functioning. People who knew me then sometimes comment on how different I am now. There's no magic involved, I tell them. I've done a lot of learning and a lot of thinking and have figured out how to get back most of those parts of my life that I value highly. In writing this book, I hope I can help you to do the same.

Each of us is unique. No one has exactly your physical makeup and life experiences. That's why I've drawn on the knowledge and experience of hundreds of people who have fibromyalgia, and the research of health care professionals and scientists, to write this book. Certain constants have emerged, but there is room for many variations on the themes you will find here. I hope you will feel encouraged to find what works best for you, and that you will resist the temptation to blame yourself if that process takes longer than you think it should.

If you've read *Fibromyalgia: A Comprehensive Approach*, you already know that my approach to managing FM emphasizes the importance of doing as much as you can for yourself. Not as much as you think you *should* do, but as much as you *can* do.

I believe we all feel better if we push toward our limits, without overdoing.

These days, I get a lot done because there's a lot I don't do. For example, I don't have things around that need to be picked up and dusted. I don't buy clothing that needs to be ironed. I like pretty things, and I know people whose homes have something to please the eye wherever you look. My home doesn't. It is functional and relatively neat, but it isn't pretty.

One could say that prettiness is one of the things FM has made me give up. I prefer to say that forgoing prettiness is one of the ways I fight back against fibromyalgia to improve the quality of my life. It is not a sign of laziness to make things as easy and uncomplicated as possible—it's a matter of modifying your life so you can be as independent and effective as you can. It is not a sign of weakness to avoid negative stress and the people and situations that cause it—you are taking positive steps to be as healthy and feel as well as you can. These are the guiding principles behind the tips in this book. I've searched out every technique that can help you spend less energy on any given task, and in any given situation.

To improve the quality of life with a chronic illness, you must have a sense of control over the condition of your own body. But fibromyalgia's changing symptoms and flare-ups make it difficult for us to predict how we will feel and what we can do on any given day. Your first step should be to learn as much as you can about the medical community's current understanding of FM. The more you know, the more you can control the condition, and the more you feel in control.

Before we go off exploring this new country where fibromyalgia has sent us to live, we should establish a common understanding of the condition and how it affects us. After we know the reasons for the difficulties we experience, we can then turn our attention to ways to overcome them.

As of the date I am writing this, no single theory explains the many facets of FM. However, most researchers are now focusing on the difference in levels of various biochemicals in the bodies of people who have fibromyalgia and those who do not. The following is an overview of the chemicals that researchers are looking at, how they are different in people with FM, and what those differences may mean in our lives. Scientific research is showing us some things we can do on our own to bring those chemicals into a favorable balance. One purpose of this book is to present those strategies to you so that you can choose which make sense to you and then try them.

Heading the list of biochemicals implicated in fibromyalgia is the neurotransmitter serotonin, which is involved in sleep, mood, and appetite. Studying serotonin in the brain is difficult; instead, researchers have measured it in the spinal fluid of people who have fibromyalgia. Two independent studies have found a lower-than-normal presence of serotonin in people with fibromyalgia. Why this is so remains a mystery. We get serotonin—and all of the chemicals in our bodies—from the food we eat. Tryptophan, one of the essential amino acids that form proteins, is the source of serotonin. When we eat foods high in tryptophan (meats, particularly lamb and turkey; carbohydrates, particularly bananas; and dairy products), some of that amino acid combines with other amino acids to make protein cells and some is used to make serotonin. The body has a mechanism that, in theory, determines how much tryptophan will be allocated to each purpose.

Just why this mechanism doesn't work properly in people with fibromyalgia is unknown. Perhaps our metabolism, the process that breaks food down into its component substances and puts them to work, is faulty. It may be that we don't absorb the food we eat efficiently, and so don't get maximum benefit from it. Or we may lack the specific enzyme that changes tryptophan into serotonin. Evidence exists to support each of these theories, but so far there's no proof.

When serotonin levels are low, we may eat more food than we need for energy, we may feel depressed, and we are likely to feel pain more intensely than we otherwise would. The chemical that signals pain is known as substance P. An elevated level of substance P causes an elevated response to pain. Researchers have found a relationship between the amounts of serotonin and substance P in human subjects: When serotonin is low, substance P is increased. An article in the journal *Arthritis and Rheumatism* reported substance P levels in the spinal fluid of people with fibromyalgia are on average three times greater than in people presumed to be healthy.[1] This finding suggests that the pain-sensing system in people who have fibromyalgia is overactive, reporting sensations as painful that others would consider innocuous. This is important information. We will return to it when we talk more about pain.

Another biochemical of interest is human growth hormone (hGH). This hormone has important functions beyond promoting normal growth in children; one is the repair throughout life of the microscopic damage muscles sustain during some kinds of normal motion. Microtears that are not repaired can cause some of fibromyalgia's pain. Most growth hormone is secreted by the pituitary gland during deep sleep; some is produced during aerobic exercise. This is another important bit of knowledge that can help us in our quest for improved quality of life.

The third biochemical that should concern us is the hormone cortisol, secreted by the adrenal gland twice a day, morning and evening. People with fibromyalgia have been found to have abnormally low levels of cortisol over a twenty-four-hour period. In some of them, releases of cortisol are too low in the morning and too high in the evening. The abnormal release pattern may explain why many of us find it hard to get going in the morning and to "shut down" at night. Cortisol helps us handle stress. Levels that are too low overall may account for how sensitive we are to stress. Some research suggests that an insufficient supply of cortisol may increase our sensitivity to pain. Stress can cause pain, and pain can certainly cause stress in a vicious cycle we will want to try to break.

Among the other chemicals that have been found to be out of balance in people with fibromyalgia, only one more—the cytokines—concerns us now in our quest to make our lives better. These immune system hormones are activated when the body is fighting illness. Cytokines are also increased in response to a lack of deep, restorative sleep. When they are given to people with cancer or multiple sclerosis as part of treatment, cytokines have been found to cause aching muscles, mental confusion, and other symptoms associated with FM. Cytokines also cause cognitive problems by interfering with the action of acetylcholine, the brain chemical associated with cognition, reasoning, and memory. We will revisit the subject of cytokines in chapter 5, on sleep.

The message to take away from this discussion is that chemical imbalances exacerbate fibromyalgia symptoms. There are things we can do to bring our body chemistry closer to a normal balance, to conserve energy, and reduce pain. The chapters that follow will present practical advice.

I address this book to people with fibromyalgia, but it's not exclusively for us. Anyone with a chronic illness, particularly anyone in chronic pain, can use the tips, techniques, and attitudes contained here. People who are normal and healthy (I call them NDAs—people Not Diagnosed with Anything) can learn from this book as well.

When I was a child, my father was a motion and time study engineer—an efficiency expert, in other words. His work involved observing people at work on an assembly line that made aircraft parts, charting their movements, and using a stopwatch to time them. The purpose of this was not to criticize the assembly line workers and get them into trouble; it was to devise better ways to get the work done with a minimum of fatigue and wasted time. A war was going on, and aircraft parts were needed to help the United States fight that war. The incentive to conserve time, energy, and materials was enormous.

After he studied and timed each process, he would think up ways to make things better for the workers by changing the way parts moved along the assembly line, suggesting improvements in seating arrangements and standing surfaces, and so forth. The word *ergonomics* hadn't been coined yet, but my efficiency-expert father knew the importance of proper support for the position of the body that was doing the work. For years he suffered from unremitting back pain that his doctor said was due to arthritis. I believe his own pain taught him the lessons we all must learn if we are to live successfully in spite of fibromyalgia.

My father brought his efficiency expert's attitudes and knowledge home with him at night. I remember him standing in the kitchen doorway and watching my sister and me as she washed and I dried the dinner dishes. I can see the kitchen now, as I write this. Kitchen counters, as we know them now, didn't exist then. There was a sink with a drainboard to the right, grooved and sloped so that water ran back into the sink. A small metal utility table on wheels stood to the left of the sink. A stove, refrigerator, and the kitchen table and chairs completed the kitchen. My sister washed and rinsed the dishes, placing them in a wire rack on the drainboard, from which I took each in turn, dried it, and put it away in the cupboard that was above the utility table. Each time I dried a glass or dish, I walked around behind my sister to the cupboard. I was younger and smaller than she in those days (I'm still younger), and I couldn't keep up with her. The dish rack would fill up, and from time to time she would have to stop and wait for me to make space for more wet dishes.

My father took this all in and came up with a plan. He moved the utility table to the right of the drainboard and told me to stack the dried dishes on it. When I was done, I rolled the table back to its regular place, directly under the cupboard, and put the dishes away all at once. That simple adjustment kept me from having to walk back and forth to the cupboard. It saved time and allowed me to keep up with my sister so we both got finished faster.

Of course, my sister and I did as my father said, but we didn't appreciate his interference right away. Once a habit is established, few people like the idea of changing it. Children are no different from adults in this way. But gradually I found myself looking for other ways to simplify the things I had to do each day: making my bed with the fewest trips around it, finding the shortest route to walk to school, the most efficient ways to put away my toys, schoolbooks, and clean laundry.

It was a game I played with myself, and I still play it. When I clear off the dinner table at night, I arrange things so I can carry more to the sink in one trip. I have a basket that goes upstairs and down with me. In it I put items I want to move from one floor to the other. I have a designated staging area on each floor—safely away from but in view of the staircase—where I put the basket when I'm on that floor. I find that a moment's thought before I do things saves me time and energy that I can put to better use in other ways. Sometimes I resent having to think about everything I do before I do it, but I know it's worthwhile. That thoughtfulness preserves my energy, letting me do more of the things I want to do.

The degree to which we can do what we want to do, to have satisfying relationships with partners and family members, to live in a home that is comfortable and nurturing, to have friends and interests outside our home, and to feel we are worthwhile members of society—these are quality-of-life issues that concern us all. Two 1993 studies measured the quality of life of women with fibromyalgia against that of women with rheumatoid arthritis, osteoarthritis, chronic obstructive pulmonary disease, insulin-dependent diabetes, and lupus.[2] In almost every category, women with FM scored lower than those with the other chronic diseases.

Improving the quality of one's life is a valid objective for anyone, particularly for anyone with fibromyalgia. To help you achieve that objective, this book looks at ways to make life easier in various settings and activities—at home, at work, and while traveling. Chapters 5 and 8 deal with sleep and nutrition, respectively, the two areas where many of us need to put most of our focus. There are suggestions throughout the book for dealing with some of the more vexing problems that often come with fibromyalgia. In chapter 10, we'll discuss standing up for yourself when dealing with doctors and health care organizations.

I've included a chapter—chapter 7—on mental and spiritual ways to combat FM, because the mind profoundly affects physical well-being. You will see how to use self-talk and how to have better dealings with the people around you. Advice will help you with the cognitive problems—memory loss, confusion, fogginess—that plague some of us all the time and all of us some of the time. This is, I think, the most important part of the book. If you can get your mental and spiritual life the way you want it to be, much of the rest will be easier by far.

The underlying theme of this book is that people with FM must learn to take charge of the situation. You already know some of the ideas in this book, but it's the ones you don't know that will change your life. By modifying your actions and attitudes, you'll find yourself living more comfortably in this new country we find ourselves in. When you have FM, the rules for getting along and the standards for success are different, but life can be just as enjoyable and rewarding.

1

Take the Pain Out of Household Activities

Handling routine household chores can be a cause of pain and frustration for anyone with fibromyalgia. Candace is a wife and mother whose whole family uses humor to deal with her FM. She recounted an example: "In the early days of my FM, my son came down the stairs one morning fumbling with the buttons on his shirt. My husband asked him what was wrong.

" 'I've got a button missing,' he answered.

" 'Well, don't tell your mother,' my husband said, 'or you'll never see *that* shirt again.' "

In most homes, housework is the first thing to fall by the wayside when fibromyalgia strikes. The repetitive motions of dusting, scrubbing, and running the vacuum cleaner are often beyond the capacity of people with FM. Reaching overhead can be painful, so even a task as trivial as changing a lightbulb may become a major issue. Tracey, a thirty-one-year-old mother of two, handles the laundry and tries to keep the house "picked up," but her husband does the heavy work. "Nothing is impossible for me," she says, "but things like vacuuming and scrubbing are quite painful. I also get extremely tired so easily."

Often a woman feels a loss of self-respect when she is unable to do the physical work of running her own household, particularly if she is at home all day. Even women who go out to work expect to be able to keep house at night or on weekends, but many find it impossible. Amy, who retired at forty-three after twenty years as a caseworker for a state social service agency, used to spend her nonworking hours in bed. "My day would end when I got out of work," she says. "I'd go right to bed and stay there until morning."

Many of the women I spoke with mentioned having found fulfillment through work before fibromyalgia entered their lives. Their sense of loss is very evident. Before becoming ill, Rose worked at a nursing home and was able to transfer a 300-pound patient from bed to wheelchair and back, despite weighing only 85 pounds herself. "I loved my job," she says. "I felt that I was doing something worthwhile for others." For Rose and others like her, whose sense of competence in the outside world is dealt a heavy blow, being unable even to do their regular housework can be especially deflating. Streamlining the work of housekeeping is an important first step toward restoring self-esteem.

Cleaning

Many of us become so discouraged trying to maintain our old standards of household cleanliness that we begin to believe we can't do anything at all. If housework woes are getting you down, perhaps a new set of standards is in order. Think about this: How clean does your home really need to be? Do people visit to look for cobwebs and dust bunnies or to see you?

Bathrooms and kitchens are important, because germs can build up there and cause illness. But the danger is nowhere near as great as the ads for disinfectant cleaning solutions would have you believe. Wiping up spots and spills as they happen, especially in those two rooms where water is easily available, is much easier than cleaning them later. Even five-year-old children can learn to wipe the bathroom sink dry after they've brushed their teeth. Approached in a positive way, small children take pride in doing such grown-up things and can develop habits that will last a lifetime.

If your household includes teens and/or other adults, they can be more of a problem. But there's still hope. Wait for a time when you feel able to control the stress you feel when asking for help, and approach the subject from the standpoint of fairness. Teens usually have an especially well-tuned sense of fair play. If you can talk about this issue without feeling defensive or vulnerable, you can appeal to that sense. After all, even if you were in perfect physical condition, it wouldn't be fair for everyone in the house to leave his or her mess for you to clean up.

Dust accumulates, even in the best-run household. You don't want to wait until people can write their names in the dust, but you don't have to chase every speck, either. Depending on where you live, dusting once a week or even less can be sufficient. Try to persuade other members of your household to leave their shoes at the door and walk around in the house in slippers or socks. (This is common practice in many parts of the world.) You'll find your floors and carpets require much less washing and vacuuming.

A cluttered house always looks dirtier than a neat one, so make it a priority to eliminate clutter. It's said that we spend the first forty years of our lives accumulating things and the second forty getting rid of them. People with FM need to act as though they are in the second phase, even if they aren't. Set aside some time, perhaps once a week, to look at what you have in a particular room or part of a room and see how much you own that you don't need, never use, and would be better off without. Every time you pick something up to dust it, consider whether it really makes you happier to have it in plain view gathering dust. If it doesn't, put it away—or give it away. Shelters for homeless people, thrift shops, and charitable organizations would love to receive items you don't want to keep. In this way you can help others while helping yourself.

When I was raising four teens (I had FM then but didn't know it), I was always looking for ways to avoid conflicts. One sore spot was their tendency to leave belongings lying around the house. Coaxing and scolding required more energy than I could spare, so I went through the common areas—living room, dining room, kitchen—and straightened up each night before I went to bed. Articles of clothing and other personal belongings I put in a big box we called the Rat Hole, which I stored in the back hallway where it was always in view, but not where anyone could trip over it. My children learned quickly where to look for missing items, and I stopped having to remind them to put things away. I also told them I would assume that anything that stayed in the Rat Hole for more than a week was something they didn't need, and I'd give it to the Goodwill store, where someone would find and appreciate it. Not too surprisingly, nothing stayed in the Rat Hole for long, and I never had to make good on that particular promise.

Although I worked full-time, I chose to keep the common areas up to my standard of cleanliness, which meant things were just clean enough so they didn't get me down. Usually a half day on the weekend was enough to accomplish this. I usually did all the laundry, but my children folded and put away their own clothes. Their bedrooms were their responsibility. My rules were these: There had to be a clear path to the door and the window, in case of fire. Beyond that, if the room was messy enough to upset me, the door was to remain closed. If the smell of a bedroom offended me, the occupant was grounded until the room was cleaned to my satisfaction. I didn't have to nag, and I rarely had to punish. What could have been a nightmare—a single mother with four teens to raise, and four years between the youngest and the oldest—was about as stress-free as such a home could be.

But what if your home has gone beyond the point where keeping it tidy and reasonably clean is possible? Perhaps you have needed to stay in bed most of the time, and you haven't had a good working relationship with those you live with in terms of cleaning up. It's not too late to remedy the situation.

It will take time, patience, and some money or creativity, but it can be done.

Start with the worst room or the sight that bothers you most. This criterion—the thing that bothers you most—is extremely important. The goal of this exercise is to make you feel better, not to win an award for Homemaker of the Year. Maybe it's the bathroom floor or dusty tabletops or the inside of the refrigerator. Pick the time of day when your energy level is at its highest or, if things are really bad for you right now, the time when your pain level is as low as it gets during the day. When that time arrives, tackle your target for the day. Do what you can for fifteen or twenty minutes, then take a five- or ten-minute break and get back to work. It may take you all day to sweep and mop the bathroom floor, but at the end of the day you'll have a clean bathroom floor and one less thing to make you miserable.

Too often we don't begin a task because we can't see how we can do it all. "Divide and conquer" should be your motto: Break the job up into pieces and do one piece. Tomorrow is another day, and you can do another piece.

Two other possibilities exist for getting your home back under control. One requires money, the other friends. If you can afford it—and it may be worth skimping on something else to do this—hire someone to come in and do a one-time cleaning. A commercial cleaning service is the ideal, but for a less costly alternative, contact the local high school or community college guidance office, which may keep a list of students looking for odd jobs. Or you might strike a barter agreement with a friend: You'll mind her children if she'll do some cleaning for you, for example. Another option is to organize a work party. Ask some friends to give you the help you need in order to whip your home into shape; in return, you provide a simple but filling meal (home-delivered pizza comes to mind, but you're probably more creative than that). Everybody wins. Your friends have a good time and a good feed, and go home knowing they've made a real difference in your well-being. You get your home back under control and can take it from there.

• • • • • Cleaning Tips • • • • •

• Use long-handled dusters to minimize reaching. Synthetic dusters are easier to clean afterward. Start by dusting the TV to build up a good static charge. Dust will then stick to the duster, and you can shake it off out a window or door when you're done for the day.

• After defrosting the freezer, spray the dry surfaces with a nonstick vegetable spray such as PAM. The next time you need to do the job, ice will drop off the freezer walls in sheets.

• To keep your hands warm when you're cleaning the refrigerator or freezer, wear knit gloves under rubber gloves. You may need to buy a larger size than usual, but it's worth the expense. If your hands get cold, soak them in lukewarm—not hot—water.

• It's usually easier to do one room at a time, rather than doing one job (such as dusting) throughout the house. If you clean one room each day, you'll have one of the cleanest homes in the neighborhood.

• Use a long-handled bath brush to clean the bathtub to eliminate kneeling and stretching.

• Pay attention to your body as you clean. If one muscle group starts aching while you're doing a chore, stop work and note where you left off. Take a short rest break and then start something new. Don't do any one activity for more than twenty minutes at a time.

• Work to music if possible. Sing if you can. (Of course you can. Nobody's listening.) Singing helps you breathe fully, and it makes the time pass faster.

• If you use fitted sheets and a comforter with a removable cover, making the bed is a matter of fluffing up the pillows and straightening out the comforter. Once a week you can wash the sheets and comforter cover and put them back on the bed, to avoid having to fold them.

• When you must lift, bend your knees slightly and keep the load close to your body.

• Pace yourself. Always stop while you can still do a bit more.

• • • • • • • • • • • • • • • • • • •

Cooking and After-Meal Cleanup

"Cooking isn't fun the way it used to be, and I can't stand long enough to cook anything that requires constant attention," Phyllis says.

For many people, preparing food for others is a way to express love for them, so losing that ability can be heartbreaking. We who have FM may need to redefine the word *meal*, trimming it from a soup-to-nuts presentation to something simpler. Fancy appetizers and desserts are unnecessary except for festive occasions. One-dish meals, perhaps with a salad on the side, are quite adequate. You can remain well nourished, and the stress of meal preparation is reduced.

When my children were in their early teens and my work brought me home at 6:00 P.M., I began dreading the words that greeted me when I opened the front door. "Hi, Mom, what's for dinner?" they'd ask, even though they had been home for three hours or so. I didn't like feeling dread—or anger or resentment—so I gave some thought to how to fix matters. The children already had rotating assignments to help clean up after dinner. I offered an amendment: Whoever cooks dinner doesn't have to clean up. Suddenly they all developed an interest in learning to cook. I was a very willing teacher.

We began planning meals on Saturday mornings. I usually

took one of the children with me in the afternoon to go shopping for whatever ingredients we needed. We all signed up on the kitchen bulletin board for the days we'd do the cooking. (One of my turns was "garbage night": leftovers I would dress up to make their encore appearance a bit different from their premiere.) Even on nights when it was my turn to cook, I was no longer asked what was for dinner the minute I came in the door; menus were posted, and anyone who was curious could check the schedule.

Sometimes a desire to avoid unpleasantness is a powerful motivator for finding a solution. At other times the motivation comes from a desire to conserve energy and minimize pain. Here are some suggestions that you might find helpful in your kitchen:

• • • • • Kitchen Setup • • • • •

• Haunt yard sales and flea markets to find a high stool, preferably with a back, to pull up to the kitchen counter during food preparation time. Alternatively, do your chopping and slicing at the kitchen table. Don't stand if you can sit.

• Try pulling out an under-the-counter drawer and putting a board across it to make a cutting board at which you can sit.

• An office secretary's chair with a lever for height adjustment may be useful in the kitchen. You can roll from refrigerator to counter to oven.

• If you must stand at the kitchen counter or sink, try placing a footstool beside you and putting one foot up on the stool. Alternate sides from time to time. It's a real back-pain reliever.

• • • • Food Preparation • • • •

• Cook foods that may be used in a variety of dishes. For example, roast a large chicken for Sunday and have chicken à la king, chicken croquettes, and chicken salad later in the week.

• Cook meals that can do double duty as leftovers. Many dishes, such as thick soups and stews, improve with age as their flavors have a chance to blend.

• Store smaller-than-meal-size quantities of leftover meats and vegetables—and the water the vegetables were cooked in—in small containers in the freezer. When you have an interesting collection, thaw and heat the items in a big pot. Add a bit of seasoning and perhaps a can of tomatoes. With just a little effort you'll have a pleasant soup.

• If you have children old enough to fend for themselves at times, declare a "You're on Your Own" night when you really need a break. Don't wait for an emergency to introduce this concept. Also, try to give them a few hours' warning so they don't have to start thinking about feeding themselves when they're already hungry. You can make it easier for your children to prepare their own meals by keeping a stock of leftovers in a designated section of the refrigerator: Cooked pasta, ground meat or turkey already browned, spaghetti sauce, cheese, and cooked rice are good to have on hand for such times.

• Use the kitchen counter as a salad bar. Put out salad greens, sliced tomatoes, sliced or grated carrots and radishes, grated cheese, thawed frozen peas, chickpeas, sprouts, raisins, nuts, cold sliced beets, and so forth. You can prepare these foods while seated at the kitchen table. Don't forget the salad dressing. (You can serve taco shells and fixings this way, too.)

• A slow cooker can be a lifesaver—if you remember to start it first thing in the morning. Meats may need to be browned first; add cut-up vegetables and a bit of water and seasoning, and your dinner will be ready when you are.

• Do your mixing and pouring in the sink or right next to it. Spills will be easier to clean up.

• If you're cooking from a recipe (not a bad idea if your brain is foggy), assemble the ingredients first and measure them all. Small quantities of dry ingredients can go onto squares of waxed paper; larger quantities and liquids go in bowls or cups. It's easier to avoid confusion if everything is in front of you when you start to cook.

• Do your cooking during your best hours. Most items can be reheated in the oven or microwave. Many foods even improve when they are reheated. Pay attention to refrigeration needs, though. Don't give bacteria a warm place to grow.

• You needn't grate cheese. Freeze hard cheese in serving portions. When it defrosts, it crumbles in your hand.

• When your hands are numb and stiff and you have to carry something filled with liquid, practice a technique used by experienced table servers: Look straight ahead, not at what you are carrying. You're much less likely to spill it if you don't look at it.

• • • • • • Cleanup • • • • • •

• Serve food directly from the pot to the plate and eliminate the need to wash serving bowls.

• If you must unload the dishwasher, take items from the machine and stack them on the counter, rather than going straight from the dishwasher to the shelf. If there's no one around to put things on the upper shelves, consider sitting on the counter while you do it.

• If you have children old enough to open the refrigerator, give them their own sports water bottles, the plastic kind with a straw built into the lid. Let it be their responsibility to keep their own bottles filled and refrigerated. They'll feel like athletes and love the independence, and you'll have fewer glasses to wash. If your children aren't in the habit of drinking water, this is a good way to encourage them to do so.

• • • • • • • • • • • • • • • • • •

Shopping for Food

For some of us, going to the supermarket is the only time we do any serious walking, which makes shopping a healthy activity. For those who find the walking involved too painful or tiring, however, some markets today provide motorized carts. If one is available where you shop and you feel you need it, don't be shy. It's there for you, not just for people who otherwise use wheelchairs. If you don't see one, perhaps that is because no one has ever expressed the need for it. You can do yourself and others a great favor by requesting that the store supply one.

Whether you're on foot or on wheels, your shopping trip will be more pleasant if you plan ahead. Make a map of the market, showing where items are shelved. Your supermarket may even have such a map available on request. If you prepare your shopping list according to where items are found in the store, you'll save energy and avoid retracing your steps. Making a shopping list before you leave home is always a good idea. Studies have shown that people with lists spend less time and money in the market than those who shop on impulse. They're less likely to forget to buy an important item, too. In my home we keep a list posted on the kitchen wall. Whoever empties a container or uses the last of an item we normally keep in stock writes it on the shopping list. That way, we keep our food and supplies inventory under control.

Laundry and Sewing

Laundry issues for people with FM involve every aspect of the job—from getting the dirty laundry to and from the laundry room and into the washer to transferring the wet laundry to the dryer to folding it and putting it away. If you look at each phase with a critical eye, you can probably solve most of the problems.

For example, if you have to get dirty clothes downstairs to the laundry room, instead of carrying the load, you might stuff it into a pillowcase or laundry bag and toss or roll it downstairs. Let gravity work for you every chance you get. If you're as apt to fall as most people with FM are, it certainly works against you often enough.

Getting the laundry back upstairs is a bit more of a problem than bringing it down. If you can't find someone to help, perhaps you need not carry it up all at once. Where wrinkles aren't a consideration (as with underwear and socks, for example), stuff items back in the pillowcase and sling it over your shoulder. If you carry a laundry basket, be sure to hold it close to your body and not out in front of you.

For Anna, the hardest part of doing laundry was getting the clothes out of the washer and into the dryer, which required her to lift heavy, wet items and bend over while holding them. Her husband relieved the strain on her sore back by putting the dryer up on cinder blocks. Something to remember anytime you're bending is to bend your knees and bend from the hips. As an Alexander Technique teacher (more about this in chapter 9) once pointed out to me, we are hinged at the hips, but not at the waist. Bending at the waist is one cause of back strain we can easily eliminate.

If you haven't thought lately about your choice of laundry products, perhaps it's time to do so. Even if you aren't susceptible to chemical and airborne allergens, ask yourself whether you really benefit from perfumed products. Nowadays, it's easy to buy unscented laundry detergents; even some major manufacturers sell them. You may find you feel better, breathe more easily, and have fewer headaches if you rid your life entirely of needlessly scented substances.

If you don't have a place in the laundry room to sit while you fold laundry, do the job at the kitchen table or sitting on the bed. If your neatness standards will allow it, consider what really must be folded and what can just be placed in the drawer. And if you have children who are old enough, let them fold their own laundry. Keep in mind that often what is a chore to an adult is a treat to a child eager to be considered capable and reliable.

Mending is another of those household tasks that often get put off to another day—a day that never comes. My sewing pile used to be a household joke until I figured out that sewing on one button or stitching one seam is easier than doing a dozen at the same time. Now my sewing basket sits beside my living room chair, and items that need attention are folded and placed on top of it. When I sit down in the evening, I usually take care of the mending first. It rarely takes more than five minutes, and when it's done that's one less thing to annoy me.

If you already have the ironing board out, iron-on patches and fusible webbing, found in most fabric and needlework shops, can come in handy. A fabric glue works well to fix seams on work and play clothes; you probably shouldn't use it on any article of clothing you really care for, but for utility clothing it's quite acceptable.

Home Modifications

You can probably look around your home and find things that can make your life easier. Ed, my husband, is not a carpenter; he doesn't even consider himself particularly handy, although I do. Nevertheless, he's done some things around our house that have made me much more independent and enabled me to feel more like a full partner in running our home and tiny farm.

When Ed built our barn (I couldn't help because I was bedridden that summer), he built a staircase to the haymow, rather than the ladder most barns have. The stairs are wide and shallow and easy for me to climb. He also built a staircase to the root cellar, where we store our winter vegetables. I don't do ladders; I'm not very well coordinated.

Because the barn is set on a hill, and getting to the door means climbing the hill and turning a right angle at the corner of the barn, he put a handrail on two sides of the barn. In winter, when it's snowy and icy, it helps me continue to do the morning chores instead of turning them over to him, which I hate to do. I really enjoy getting outside at dawn every day and feeding our sheep and chickens. The chicken coop is also up a hill from the house. My husband built a set of stairs into the hill with railroad ties and bricks so I don't have to try to get up the hill itself.

Finally, my office is on the ground level of our house; the bathroom is up a flight of stairs. I want stairs between me and the bathroom. It gives me more exercise than I'd get if everything were on one floor. But the typical staircase is too steep for me to handle in comfort. Ed rebuilt the staircase, making the steps wider and more shallow and thus easier to climb.

Once you have adopted the habit of examining your routine household activities with a critical eye, you will probably think of many more adjustments to add to those in this chapter. If you do, and are willing to share them, I'd be happy to hear from you.

2

Maximize Moments of Pleasure

We all need moments of pleasure and joy in our lives. Some people who have fibromyalgia give up their favorite activities when pain interferes. But with planning, you can make modifications that allow you to participate in most of your chosen leisure activities. The tips in this chapter are organized around gardening and entertaining; however, you can adapt them to other pursuits.

The time you invest in doing things you enjoy can brighten your outlook and give pleasure to those around you as well. You may find you need to adjust your standards of performance, but no one expects you to be perfect. In this chapter you will find ideas that will inspire you to bring zest back to your life.

Gardening
....

Approached thoughtfully, mindful of our physical limitations, gardening can make a tremendous contribution to the quality of our lives. Fresh vegetables, grown without chemical poisons, harvested with care, and consumed while they are still chock full of nutrients, nourish the body. Flowers provide beauty and nourish the soul. Done correctly, gardening provides exercise and enhances our sense of well-being.

Robert, a disabled nurse, says, "I've had to modify the way I approach gardening in recent years—no more all-day marathons that knock me down for the following week." Still, he adds, "Most years I can grow and preserve enough to feed my family year round." Robert bases his gardening technique on the popular book *Square Foot Gardening,* by Mel Bartholomew (Rodale Press). "The basic principle," Robert explains, "is to grow in small, intensively planted sections, each section the same size as the others, and the soil in each section nurtured and fed to maintain the health, structure, and fertility necessary to support the heavy plantings."

Each bed is sized so that Robert can reach any part of it while sitting on the ground or kneeling on a padded kneeling bench. Rows are spaced just wide enough for a weeder with a four-inch blade. "Whether the task is planting, weeding, feeding, or harvesting, I can complete the entire bed in five to ten minutes. If I can only do one or two beds in a session, that's OK, because I know that I have completed an entire bed and have some sense of accomplishment. I do a couple of beds in the morning, a few in the afternoon or evening, and they get more care and attention than they would if I had made big beds or long rows. I would never get through a single bed in a whole day, and I probably wouldn't even try."

Flora specializes in growing flowers and uses an informal style she calls "cottage gardening." "It doesn't require firm rules, straight lines, formal plantings, and well-weeded beds," she explains. She places large rocks, twelve to eighteen inches high, as accents. More important, she points out, the rocks are a place to sit while she weeds the surrounding areas. She chooses perennial plants (the kind that grow back year after year) rather than annuals (which last only one year). Plants on sale at garden and farm stands are usually tagged as annuals or perennials.

She suggests placing plants much closer together than the seed packets and gardening books recommend. "The goal is to cover every inch of ground," says Flora. "Space plants at half the distance recommended in gardening books. Weeds cannot grow on ground covered by plants." She also recommends using an organic mulch such as wood chips to cover the bare ground until plants grow to full size.

Flora recommends having a compost pile, "not so much for the compost, but as an easy place to dispose of weeds and plants you have trimmed. Hide it behind a U-shaped planting of bushes, where no one can see it. Make sure it has easy access so you can just push your wheelbarrow up to it and dump."

Alana, who lives in Alaska, grows her vegetables in beds raised about eighteen inches off the ground. "I can sit on the edge and reach everything," she says. "Not only do the plants grow better because the soil stays warmer, which is important in our climate. Also we don't have any slugs, and we get fewer weeds."

Gardens don't have to be large to be enjoyable. Hanging planters and whiskey barrels cut in half lengthwise and placed on their sides make attractive containers for small spaces. Flora suggests filling the containers half full with those foam peanuts you've been wondering how to get rid of, and the rest with soil.

Alana describes her routine for reducing muscular pain when she gardens. She stretches gently before starting and takes a half-dose of muscle relaxant and painkiller. "I use enough to keep me from getting into awkward positions because I'm guarding sore areas—that would make it worse later—but not so much that I won't know immediately when it's time to stop," she says. She also takes frequent breaks to stretch. When she's done in the garden, she takes a long, hot bath and rests the remainder of the day, doing very mild stretching exercises periodically.

• • • • • Gardening Tips • • • • •

• Move slowly. Make gardening a time for relaxation and meditation. Think about what you are doing and not about how much you want to get done. Gardening can be a wonderful spirit booster, but only if you let it be. If it becomes a painful, burdensome obligation, it's time to stop.

• Invest in the best, most ergonomically designed tools you can find. Gardening supply catalogs are increasingly paying attention to the fact that some people have sore hands and backs, and are providing tools that make the work easier.

• Especially useful is a kneeling bench. Placed one way, it serves as a seat. Turned upside down, it is a padded kneeler. The tubular legs that support the bench become handholds to help you when you stand up.

• Bring a water bottle to the garden and drink frequently. If you wait until you're thirsty, you're already partly dehydrated. Symptoms of dehydration include fatigue and shakiness. Dehydration is easy to avoid.

• If you're gardening in rocky soil, use levers to pry out rocks and then roll them out of the way. It's amazing how much you can do without lifting if you think about it.

• When you're finished in the garden, lie down on your stomach for about fifteen minutes and concentrate on relaxing the muscles in your back. Most back problems start after the work is done and the muscles cramp up, not while you're actually doing the work.

• • • • • • • • • • • • • • • • •

Entertaining

Maintaining an active social life when you have fibromyalgia is nearly impossible. Standing for long periods, as one is apt to do at a party, hurts too much to be worth the effort. If you're avoiding alcohol and sweets, it's hard to spend hours among people who have no similar restrictions. The practice of good sleep hygiene, which includes being in bed at the same time each night, makes Cinderella seem like a night owl compared to you.

You find yourself regretfully declining invitations until the invitations stop coming. Even if your friends understand, they're apt to see no point in inviting you when they know you won't come. They may even think it would be unkind to remind you of a party that you can't attend. Still, it hurts to be left out.

Even worse, you've probably given up inviting friends to visit. Entertaining seems too challenging when you're not feeling well. It probably seems that way because you're using your old standards, the ones you had before you developed fibromyalgia. It's time to rethink those standards and adopt new ones that will allow you to have a social life, even if it's not the one you used to have.

Invite people because you want to see them, not out of a sense of obligation. Think small: A group of six lets everyone find a place to sit. Let the music set the mood; you don't want things to be too stimulating, so play soft music quietly and keep the lights on fairly low. Food should be plentiful, but it doesn't have to be elaborate. Most people genuinely enjoy pot-luck suppers, where everyone contributes. Let your guests choose what they'll bring, but ask them to tell you so you don't wind up with two main dishes and no dessert.

It takes only one good conversationalist to keep a group of six engaged, and that one person doesn't have to be you. However, it is a good idea to have a couple of topics in mind to get the talk rolling, especially if the people you invite don't know each other. The key here is to invite people who have something in common.

I once invited three couples (and their children) for Sunday brunch. I was the only person who knew them all, but I thought they'd click. That's what I told them all: that there were some other people I thought they should know, and that I'd leave it to them to find out why. The gathering was such a success that it lasted from noon until 8:00 P.M., and ended then only because the children had to be put to bed. The food I served for brunch was simple and prepared ahead of time. For the rest of the day I gave everyone permission to look in the cupboards and refrigerator when they wanted anything. When we got hungry again late in the afternoon and nobody wanted to go home, we raided the pantry and put together a rather imaginative spaghetti supper, with everyone helping to cook and clean up. The day was tiring for me, but exhilarating, and led to many more such gatherings in each of our homes.

The Holidays Need Not Be a Pain

For many people who have fibromyalgia, all the feelings of being left out and unable to participate fully in a social life come into sharpest focus during the holiday season. Thanksgiving Day, Christmas, Hanukkah, Kwanzaa, New Year's Eve, and New Year's Day can provide bitter reminders of all the things expected of us, and all the things we cannot do.

Houseguests arrive, party invitations come in the mail, gifts must be purchased and delivered. There are cookies to bake, cards to sign and address, decorations to put up, and a host of other commitments to be met. It all seems so impossible that it's no wonder the winter holiday season is often more stressful than pleasurable. Even people who don't have FM feel the pressure, but for those who do have it, developing strategies to get through the holidays is essential.

• • • • • Holiday Tips • • • • •

• If houseguests are inevitable, help them to be self-sufficient. Show them where towels, dishes, and other necessities are kept and encourage them to help themselves. Before your guests' arrival, mark clearly those food items in the refrigerator that are off-limits because you have special plans for them; then tell your guests to feel free to eat everything else.

• Don't try to prepare three meals a day. Tell your guests what time you'll serve dinner, and suggest that they plan to take care of themselves for breakfast and lunch. They will probably feel more at home if they are encouraged to fend for themselves some of the time.

• Keep to your normal sleep schedule; it is the most important thing you can do for yourself. You can't sit up chatting all night and expect to function the next day. Tell your guests that you have this need and excuse yourself. Don't draw a lot of attention to your leave-taking by apologizing or voicing regret about missing out on the rest of the evening. Making a fuss about your bedtime will make your guests uncomfortable.

• Don't give up your bed to a guest. That's what sofa beds and guest rooms are made for.

• Cook ahead and freeze as much as you can. There is no virtue in doing things the hard way. Look at every task with a critical eye, and figure out the easiest way to do it. Cut corners wherever possible.

• If it's up to you to host the holiday dinner, consider having at least some of it catered or making the dinner a potluck event. Your guests would rather have a host who enjoys having them come to dinner than one who makes them feel guilty by being too tired to be able to enjoy the meal and their company.

• Watch what you eat. Nutrition is just as important to your health at this time of the year as at any other. Don't skip meals and make up for it in snacks.

• If you've got your sugar intake under control (as you should if you want to feel your best), summon all the self-control you can when goodies are within reach. If you are going to a party where guests contribute food items, bring something sugar-free to be sure you have something to eat.

• Alcohol interferes with slow wave, deep sleep—the kind of sleep that people with FM find so elusive. Before you lift that glass, think about whether it is worth the price. Make decisions that affect your health; don't let yourself get swept along with the tide.

• Discover mail-order catalogs. Lots of companies accept telephone orders for Christmas delivery until about December 22. Many catalogs offer as broad a range of items and styles as the stores in the mall do. You don't have to settle for what little information the catalog gives, either. Good mail-order companies provide toll-free phone numbers and order takers with information that can help you make your choices. For example, if you want to order a pair of slacks and the catalog doesn't list the inseam measurement, call and ask. Many companies will provide swatches on request. Any reputable mail-order company will accept returns after the holidays, provided you have kept the receipt.

• Don't fall prey to that common fear of giving a gift that the recipient will not like. Do the best you can, and let it go at that.

• Be selective about parties. Accept only those invitations that really appeal to you, and where you know the host will consider your needs and comfort. Think hard about attending evening events two nights in a row or more than one event per evening.

• Avoid situations that are raucous and overstimulating. Leave the party while you're still having a good time. Give yourself time to unwind before you try to sleep.

• If you choose not to accept any invitations, or don't get any that are appropriate for your needs, consider having a party yourself. Make it a potluck brunch or early-evening event. Playing soothing background music will tip off your guests that boisterousness is not appropriate.

• • • • • • • • • • • • • • • • •

Many people, not only those with fibromyalgia, experience feelings of loss or disappointment at holiday time. If the holiday blues get to you, write about your feelings or discuss them with your favorite good listener. Accept your feelings as normal and move on. You are not here to live up to other people's expectations. Be clear about your limitations and needs—with yourself and also with others. Avoid people who are toxic to you; surround yourself with those who are good to and for you, and enjoy yourself. Put your own needs first this year. Sometimes it is more blessed to receive than to give.

3

Strategies at Work

Companies organized to take into account the physical problems and needs of employees are rare. Most managers prefer not to know about employees' personal problems. Coworkers are understandably wary of people who complain of chronic illness—they may worry about being asked to take on additional duties without any compensating adjustment to their workload or pay. Meanwhile, most of us who are lucky enough to be able to hold a job, whether by choice or necessity, are confronted almost daily by the fact that some things that are easy for most people are difficult for us.

Accommodations on the Job

The Americans with Disabilities Act (ADA) requires U.S. employers to make "reasonable accommodations" for "a qualified individual with a disability." You are a "qualified individual" if you can perform the essential functions of your job with or without reasonable accommodations. If you have a written job description, it defines the essential functions of your job. If not, your employer's judgment of the job's essential functions will probably prevail in a dispute. The catchall phrase "and other tasks as assigned," often included in a job description, does not constitute an essential function.

A disability in ADA terms is any physical or mental impairment that substantially limits one or more of your major life activities. The inability to lift more than ten pounds or sit for more than twenty minutes, for example, satisfies this requirment even though you are not disabled. "Reasonable accommodations" include making existing facilities readily accessible to and usable by individuals with disabilities, job restructuring, providing part-time or modified work schedules, and acquiring or modifying equipment used to perform the work, among other things. If you work on an assembly line, rotating assignments so that you don't have to use the same muscles in the same pattern of movement all day long would be a reasonable accommodation.

Companies with fewer than fifteen employees are not required to comply with the ADA. Even larger companies may be excused from providing an accommodation if it causes an undue hardship, such as an unreasonable expense in view of the company's financial resources. Even if they are not required to comply, however, most employers readily see the value of providing accommodations to a loyal, experienced employee. This is a point for you to stress if you are meeting resistance in obtaining accommodations: It's cheaper to help an experienced employee stay on the job than to undertake the expense of hiring and training a new one. For small companies that have annual revenues of less than $1 million, the ADA grants a tax credit for expenditures made in the interest of access to people with disabilities. If you work for a small company, you might want to obtain Internal Revenue Service form 8826 (available at regional IRS offices and on the World Wide Web) and attach it to your written request, explaining that the employer can complete the form to claim the tax credit.

One woman with FM brought to work a note from her doctor saying that since stress makes the condition worse, she should be allowed to avoid stressful tasks. When she asked that the letter be placed in her personnel file, the director of human resources countered that every job in the company involved stress, and that if the woman couldn't handle stress the company had no suitable job for her.

A better approach is to ask the doctor for a note that specifically states which aspects of your job require accommodations. For example, the doctor might say you should not be required to work overtime or lift items weighing more than a specific amount (unless your job consists primarily of lifting). The note should also say what you can do, and should relate your abilities to the essential functions of your job, leaving no doubt about your eligibility for accommodations. You should give the doctor a list of things you believe you can and cannot do, to make it easier for her or him to write the note. You will, of course, keep a copy for yourself.

The Job Accommodation Network (JAN) provides a list of possible accommodations for people with fibromyalgia. (The network is a service of the President's Committee on Employment of People with Disabilities. See its listing in the "Resources" section.) This list is meant only to suggest possibilities, not to prescribe for specific situations, which should be evaluated on an individual basis. You can use it to stimulate your thinking if you plan on asking your employer for specific accommodations.

Attendance Issues
    Provide flexible leave for health problems
    Allow the employee to work from home
      Offer a part-time work schedule
      Provide a self-paced workload and flexible hours
    Allow sick leave to be used without penalty, family
        medical leave if eligible, or leave without pay when
        no other options are available

Fatigue-Related Issues
    Permit flexible scheduling and use of leave time
    Allow longer or more frequent rest breaks

Reduce the workload or provide a self-paced workload

Furnish job-sharing opportunities

Provide an area where the person can take rest breaks and
lie down if necessary

Allow the employee to work from home for part of the day

Reduce or eliminate physical exertion on the job

Evaluate the ergonomics of the employee's workstation

Muscle Pain and Stiffness Related Issues

Provide an accessible work environment (ramps, parking,
etc.)

Allow breaks for walking around the work environment

Provide an adjustable-height workstation to allow
alternating between sitting and standing position

Provide ergonomic chair and workstation suited to the
individual

Reduce repetitive tasks or interrupt the tasks with other
duties

Stress, Depression, and Anxiety Related Issues

Start stress management training in the workplace

Allow flexible leave to meet with counselors or physicians

Provide peer support and mentoring

Chronic Headache-Related Issues

Permit flexible scheduling

Reduce visual and auditory distractions

Adjust lights in the working environment by providing
task lighting, filtering or dimming fluorescent
lighting, or using full-spectrum lighting

Control contrast on the computer monitor, using a glare
guard

Provide proper ventilation of the work area, possibly
adding air-purification devices

Concentration-Related Issues

Reduce visual and auditory distractions by isolating the

work environment, using environmental sound
machines or sound-absorbent baffles or partitions
Increase natural lighting or provide full-spectrum lighting
Allow the employee to work from home
Plan for uninterrupted work time
Allow for frequent rest breaks
Divide large assignments into smaller tasks
Restructure the job to include only essential functions
Provide clear, written job instructions, deadlines, and
expectations
Use lists, calendars, and memory aids (electronic
organizers) to note things to be done

Bowel and Bladder Control Issues
Provide a clear, unobstructed pathway to the rest room
Allow the employee to be situated close to a rest room
Do not penalize the employee for time spent in the rest
room
Provide flexible leave for health problems

Temperature Sensitivity and Respiratory Issues
Redirect air-conditioning and heating vents
Allow the individual to wear layered clothing
Provide a portable space heater
Give the employee his/her own office with temperature
controls
Provide good ventilation and/or a portable air-purification
device
Allow the employee to work from home

Another ADA provision makes it unlawful to harass a person
because of a medical condition. If, for example, a doctor says
you need physical therapy and the only time treatment is available to you is during working hours, your employer may not
punish you in any way for taking time off for this purpose.
However, you may have to take those hours as sick leave or
personal time. An employer cannot be required to pay you, but

The following senarios, drawn from materials provided by the Job Accommodation Network, describe real-life situations and the suggested accommodations:

• *An administrative assistant for a utility company has FM. Her duties include typing, answering the telephone, and taking written messages. She reports neck pain and upper-body fatigue.* Accommodations might include using a telephone headset to reduce the pain of tilting her head and lifting her arm repeatedly, a portable angled writing surface to take written messages, and a copy holder and arm supports to be employed while typing.

• *A nurse working in a county health clinic was recently diagnosed with fibromyalgia. She typically works the evening shift, but her doctor recommends a change in shift so she can regulate her sleep patterns. She experiences a great deal of fatigue and body ache.* Accommodations might include changing from evening shift to day shift, spreading shifts out rather than working two twelve-hour shifts back to back, reducing the number of hours worked or offering part-time work as an option, and permitting rest breaks whenever possible.

• *A guidance counselor for a large high school experiences severe bouts of irritable bowel syndrome, depression, and fatigue because of fibromyalgia. He has his own office, but the office is not near a rest room. He has reported difficulty with entering the school because the front doors are too heavy for him.* Accommodations might include moving his office to a location close to and with a clear pathway to the rest room; removing the problem with the front door by adding an automatic entry system, lowering the door pressure to less than five pounds, or setting up a doorbell system that would ring in the main office and signal another employee to help him with the door;

and allowing him flexible leave time to see his therapist as needed.

• *A factory worker is experiencing decreased stamina, difficulty standing and sitting for long periods, and sensitivity to cold temperatures. Her job requires that she assemble small plastic parts as they come down a conveyor line that is approximately waist high. She typically stands to perform this function, and her station is close to an air-conditioning vent.* Accommodations might include allowing her to use a stool so that she can sit, stand, or lean while assembling parts; placing her on a part of the line that does not require a quick pace or extensive physical exertion, redirecting air-conditioning vents away from her work area, and giving her a portable space heater.

negative letters to your file, adverse comments, or additional work assignments to be done after normal working hours are all violations of the ADA.

What do you do if such a thing happens to you or if your employer ignores your request for accommodations? First, you must be sure that you have done everything required of you to qualify as a person with a disability. This means obtaining from your doctor a detailed list of the specific things you can and cannot do, as well as a statement of needed treatment and the reason it must be carried out during business hours, if you need time off from work to get that treatment. You will have to submit a written request, also in considerable detail, for the accommodations you are seeking. Since you are the person with the problem, you will probably also have to provide the solution—a list of articles to be purchased, one or more suppliers of each item, and the cost of each, if possible. Furnishing this information is not a requirement of the ADA. It's simply the most practical way to overcome your company's objections and inertia, and to get what you need so you can continue working.

The ADA provides specific remedies for those whose rights under the law have been violated, but gentle persuasion backed up by facts and medical opinion is a much better option. There are agencies to which you can turn if your request for accommodation is denied, and court action is possible. However, legal action is expensive and time-consuming; the net effect on the quality of your life is unlikely to be beneficial. If they have a backlog of requests for assistance, ADA agencies usually give preference to people with obvious disabilities such as blindness or a missing limb. Expect to be your own advocate in ADA matters. You may get help from the personnel department or the employee assistance program, but here, as in most matters relating to fibromyalgia, you cannot depend on the kindness of strangers.

The most common occupational hazards for office workers, not only those with fibromyalgia, are back pain and repetitive strain injury. With the heightened pain sensitivity of FM, you are more likely than your coworkers to experience these problems, but you need not claim accommodations under the ADA to reduce the risks associated with desk work, particularly work involving a computer. The following sections deal with ways to make your work life more livable.

Sitting for Your Living

Your chair is the most important piece of equipment in your office. Your employer should be eager to see that you have proper seating. Without it, you can't possibly do your best work, and that's what you were hired to do. If you are the only person who sits in your chair, you will probably have to adjust it only occasionally. If you work in different chairs, or if someone else uses your chair on a different shift, you'll need to make adjustments more frequently. Learn which chair settings are the best for you, marking them with tape, if necessary, so you won't have to use trial and error each time you sit down to work.

You should be able to adjust the seat's height, the height and angle of the back rest, and the angle of the seat. The seat should be high enough to allow your thighs to be approximately parallel to the floor while your feet rest flat on the floor. A footrest, preferably angled up toward the toes, may be necessary if your feet can't rest comfortably on the floor. The chair back should be placed so that it supports the curve in the small of your back. The depth of the chair should permit you to sit all the way back to take full advantage of the backrest, particularly its low-back support. If your work involves mainly reading or writing on your desktop, you may find it comfortable to tip the seat front up a bit so that more of your weight rests against the back of the seat. If you work mainly on a computer and find yourself leaning forward, make the seat slope slightly downward at the front so that it doesn't dig into the backs of your thighs. Your chair should have armrests that support your elbows. Depending on the kind of work you are doing, your forearms should be held at an angle between 75 and 90 degrees to your upper arms, and your wrists should not be flexed as you work.

The chair's swivel mechanism and casters should work smoothly. Use the swivel capability to move your whole body to face your task, rather than twisting in the chair. Don't swivel, though, to lift heavy objects such as reference books and catalogs off a shelf. Instead, lift these things from a standing position. Chairs may be equipped with four or five casters; if you have the choice, get the five-caster type. It is more stable and less likely to tip over if you move quickly.

Arrange the tools you use according to the frequency with which you use them. Picture your work surface as divided into two curved zones. The first is the high-priority zone, a half-moon shape whose far edge is the farthest you can reach without leaning forward or stretching. In this area you should place only those items you use frequently. The low-priority zone is an arc six to eight inches beyond the half-moon. It holds items you use only infrequently. Rarely used objects should be stored on shelves above or away from your desk. I keep some things I use often, but not when I'm concentrating, at a distance from my desk. In this way I make myself stand up and move around more often than I would if everything were within reach.

Making myself move this way is my variation of the advice that people with fibromyalgia should never sit still for more than twenty minutes at a time. We stiffen if we sit longer than that. However, it takes most people about fifteen minutes to get to the point of peak concentration, so if your work requires you to focus, the twenty-minute rule isn't practical. I become stiff from sitting, so before I get up after a long work session, I shift about in my chair and try to loosen things up. After a moment of stretching, standing up isn't nearly as painful. When it's not necessary for me to concentrate intensely, I stand up quite often to make up for the periods of inactivity.

Repetitive Strain Injury

If your work requires you to stay in a fixed position, repeating the same motions for long periods, you are a candidate for a repetitive strain injury (RSI). If you have been ignoring pain in your hand, wrist, arm, neck, shoulder, or back, perhaps telling yourself it is merely one more nuisance associated with fibromyalgia, you should seek medical attention immediately. Perhaps you're right, but you should not assume so because the damage done by unremitting repetitive motion with insufficient time to rest and recover can be irreversible.

RSI is one of several terms for a cumulative trauma disorder (CTD). Other names are repetitive motion disorder (RMD) and repetitive motion injury (RMI). RSI includes a range of diseases, including tendinitis of the hand or wrist, epicondylitis ("tennis elbow"), carpal tunnel syndrome, cubital tunnel syndrome, and thoracic outlet syndrome. Office workers get most of the attention when RSI is discussed, but they are not the only people subject to the ravages of repetitive motion. Stitchers, weavers, quilters, assembly workers, supermarket checkout-counter clerks, long-distance drivers, and musicians are all vulnerable. What they have in common is the requirement that they stay in the same position and do the same things repeatedly. Not only does this repetitive motion cause damage to the tendons, muscles, nerves, and joints due to friction, but also the worker's lack of body movement impedes the flow of blood to the damaged tissues, reducing the rate at which the body repairs them. Reducing the number of repetitive motions involved in your work may not be possible, but you can usually improve the blood supply to the tissues by reducing the stress of faulty posture and by engaging frequently in stretching exercises. If you have a job that requires repetitive motion, consider these as preventive measures even if you don't have symptoms of RSI.

There is good reason to suppose that people with fibromyalgia are especially susceptible to RSI. We tend to be subject to muscle spasms, which involve constricting the flow of blood and therefore of oxygen to the affected muscles. Various studies have found that people with fibromyalgia often have insufficient oxygen in their blood and tissues, including the brain. We may have problems with our posture, compounded by the unconscious effort to "guard" painful places on our bodies by adjusting our position to reduce discomfort, a tactic that places additional stress on another part of the body. Also, most of us are in terrible physical condition due to inactivity. Our muscles tighten even more, movement causes microscopic muscle tears, and a deficiency in growth hormone slows the normal process of repair.

The primary warning signals of RSI are the following:

- pain at the base of your thumb or in your wrist
- tingling and numbness in arms, hands, or fingers

- decreased strength in your grip
- loss of motor control, clumsiness
- feeling of fatigue or heaviness in your hands and forearms
- pain in your neck, back, or shoulders.

Other signs of impending problems include a heightened awareness of one or both hands; doing things with your non-dominant hand that you used to do with your dominant hand; using arms, feet, or shoulders instead of hands to open doors; and giving up customary activities or hobbies because they make your hands hurt.

RSI sneaks up on you. People often ignore their symptoms until they have had at least one episode of severe, incapacitating pain. If you have experienced any of these symptoms, even if you don't have them now, you should be checked for RSI. To ignore such injury is a great risk. Even a day or two can make the difference between a readily treatable condition and permanent damage.

Choosing a doctor to see if you suspect you have repetitive strain injury is a tricky matter. If you have a primary care physician whom you trust, that is the place to start. Specialists who see RSI patients include a physiatrist (doctor of physical medicine), neurologist, occupational medicine doctor, rheumatologist, hand surgeon, and orthopedist. Be aware, though, that hand surgeons and most orthopedists are oriented toward surgery and may recommend that option before trying anything else. Rheumatologists and orthopedists know about bones and joints, but they may know little about soft-tissue injuries and may overlook important clues.

Talk to others who have repetitive strain problems before selecting a doctor. Look for a center that deals with occupational medicine or one that focuses on musicians or athletes. If you are within phoning distance of a conservatory of music or a university that trains musicians, inquire there. If your injury is work related, you need a doctor who accepts workers' compensation cases. Ask about that before you make an appointment. You need a doctor who will be prepared to advocate for you with your employer or insurance company.

You especially want a doctor who "believes in" repetitive strain injuries *as well as fibromyalgia*. RSI is not FM, and it shouldn't be dismissed as such without a thorough examination that rules out any of the other potential problems that accompany cumulative trauma. Your repetitive strain injury may hurt worse because of your fibromyalgia. On the other hand, if you're lucky, your FM may have made you more aware of the injury at its onset. You may stand a better chance than others of recovering fully, but only if you deal with the problem promptly and follow your recommended treatment through to the end.

A note here about carpal tunnel syndrome (CTS): It is not the only kind of repetitive strain injury, nor even the most common. Do not accept a quick diagnosis of CTS, particularly if the doctor recommends surgery. Exercise, physical therapy, and modification of activities at work and at home may all lead to improvement. Be mindful, too, that you may have more than one repetitive injury. Muscles, tendons, nerves, and joints can all be involved.

Hands, arms, and backs are not the only parts of the body that are subject to RSI. Necks are vulnerable, too. Having your terminal screen at the proper level is important; the center of the screen should be at or slightly below eye level when you are looking straight ahead. If you have to tilt your head upward to see your monitor, you're headed for trouble.

A common practice of people who do a lot of work on the telephone is to cradle the telephone handset between the head and shoulder. If you do this, you should stop it now. Necks aren't meant to bend sideways, and the possibility of compressing a nerve that way is great. If you have to type while talking on the phone, your employer should give you a telephone headset that leaves both hands free.

People who have RSI must keep in mind that it developed over months or years. It will not go away in a week or two. As part of your therapy, you will probably have to endure a period of rest, which means refraining from the activities that caused the injury (such as using a computer) or that make your symptoms worse. You can expect a course of physical therapy, including deep-tissue massage and a routine of stretching and strengthening exercises that you will perform at home every day.

Fibromyalgia may have already taught you the necessity of being actively involved in decisions pertaining to your own treatment. That lesson will stand you in good stead if you must be treated for RSI. As with FM, there is little agreement among doctors about effective treatment for repetitive strain injuries. Be prepared to tolerate some more trial and error. Patience is necessary, but let your instincts tell you whether a particular therapy is helping. Don't hesitate to tell your doctor if you're not seeing improvement or if something is making you feel worse. Your doctor should value your feedback and either adjust the treatment or reassure you, explaining why it's best to continue it.

Your doctor may or may not prescribe a splint for your wrist, depending on the nature of the injury, but you should not prescribe a splint for yourself. Splints can make things worse by resting some muscles and overtaxing others. Splints prescribed for carpal tunnel syndrome are worn only at night, to keep you from flexing your wrists in your sleep. If your doctor prescribes a splint, make sure you know what the splint is supposed to accomplish and understand the instructions for wearing it.

Analgesic drugs such as aspirin, acetaminophen, and nonsteroidal anti-inflammatory drugs (NSAIDs; for example, ibuprofen and naproxen) may help with the pain, but you should use them sparingly and watch out for side effects. NSAIDs and aspirin can cause stomach upset and bleeding, particularly when taken on an empty stomach. NSAIDs are also implicated in some cases of kidney impairment. If you take these drugs and experience water retention, stop taking them and tell your doctor about it. Acetaminophen has the fewest adverse side effects, but recently evidence has emerged suggesting it should not be taken by anyone who drinks alcohol. You should not take acetaminophen while you are taking aspirin or an NSAID, nor should you take aspirin and NSAIDs concurrently.

Some people with RSI find relief in alternative treatments such as acupuncture and spinal manipulation (done by a chiropractic or osteopathic physician). However, RSI is too potentially serious to trust these methods alone. If you have a repetitive strain injury, you need both to heal it and to learn how to prevent its recurrence. Neither acupuncture nor spinal manipulation can help in this area.

Good nutrition can be helpful in relieving your RSI. Eating a diet rich in whole, unprocessed foods is a good thing for anyone to do, but you also may want to think about specific supplements (not as a substitute for good nutrition). A diet rich in refined sugar, including as little as one alcoholic beverage a day, can lead to a deficiency in the B-complex vitamins, particularly vitamin B_6. I have known several people diagnosed with carpal tunnel syndrome whose symptoms disappeared when they eliminated sugar and alcohol from their diets and took 100 mg of B_6 for three or four weeks. Don't take B_6 alone for long or you'll risk developing some other B vitamin deficiency. If you want to continue, after about three weeks you should switch to a B-complex preparation containing a similar amount of B_6. Vitamin C helps heal wounds, so it may help with a repetitive strain injury. If you smoke, you owe yourself 75 mg of vitamin C for every cigarette just to stay even. Take more than that for healing purposes. People under prolonged stress may also be deficient in vitamin C. Finally, vitamin E has been shown to minimize muscle damage and inflammation resulting from exercise, so taking 400 to 800 international units of vitamin E a day to help promote healing may be beneficial.

If you spend much of your time using a computer, the following checklist can help you evaluate the conditions under which you work. It can help you to list accommodations for which to ask your employer. Note, however, that this list applies as much to people who don't have RSI as to those who do. It is a means of preventing injury, and your employer should take it seriously, from both a human and an economic standpoint. Workers who are comfortable and free of pain are more productive by far than those who labor under adverse conditions. Approach your conversation with your employer as though it were purely a business matter, something it is in his or her best interests to attend to. You are not a supplicant and don't need to feel defensive. Go into the meeting with the attitude that you have information that will help the company get the maximum value out of its investment in you.

Checklist for Computer Work

Posture and chair

Does your working position allow you to:

- rest your feet fully on the floor or a footrest?

- bend your knees at approximately a right angle?

- sit with your thighs parallel to the floor without pressure from your chair on the backs of your thighs?

- sit with your upper body straight and your lower back well supported?

- hold your upper arms straight down close to your sides, elbows bent at right angles, and lower arms parallel to the floor?

- work with your wrists straight, bent neither up nor down, nor to the left or right?

Desk and keyboard

Can you:

- adjust the height of the desk or table so that you can view the monitor without bending or stretching your neck?

- sit with your legs comfortably under the desktop?

- keep on the desktop all the things you need in order to do your work comfortably and efficiently?

- put the keyboard at lower than desktop height so that you don't have to bend your arms upward to reach it?

- reach the shift and function keys without strain?

- tell from a decrease in pressure or an audible click when you have pressed a key hard enough for the character to appear on the screen?

Vision and lighting

Do you:

- have a way to place information you are working with on a copy stand about the same distance from your eyes as the monitor?

- have the ability to block reflections of windows or lights from reaching the screen?

- have window shades or blinds to reduce glare?

- have adequate lighting to read from documents when overall room light is too low?

- have a monitor that flickers or on which the image is blurry?*

- need to squint to read what's on the screen?*

Working conditions

Does your company:

- assign you a variety of duties, some of which don't require you to use the computer?

- set a quota that you must meet, such as a certain number of keystrokes per hour?*

- monitor your work electronically?*

- use the results to pressure you to work faster?*

- allow a break of at least fifteen minutes after two hours of computer use?

- allow you to get up and move around at will?

- teach you how to adjust your chair, desk, and monitor?

- teach and encourage you to exercise to reduce tension and muscle fatigue?

*"Yes" is the desirable answer except for questions followed by an asterisk. A "yes" answer to those questions or a "no" answer to the others gives you clues to the things that need to change if you are to improve the quality of your working life.

I've also provided some tips to make your time at the computer or office desk more comfortable (see below). For those of you who are teachers and others who have to write on wall-mounted boards, shoulder strain can be a problem. You can relieve this strain by cradling the elbow of the hand that does the writing in the palm of the nondominant hand. Keep both elbows close to your body and walk, don't reach, as you write.

● ● ● ● ● ● ● ● ● ● ● ● ● ● ● ● ●
Tips for Making Computer Work More Comfortable

- To support your wrists at the keyboard, fold a hand towel three or four times and put it in front of the keyboard.

• Your mouse should be up against the keyboard on the side of your dominant hand with a pad made of a folded washcloth to elevate your wrist there as well.

• Use your fingers, not your shoulder, to move the mouse. Be sure your arm is supported, not hanging in the air from your shoulder while you use the mouse.

• Learn as many keystroke equivalents as you can to minimize the use of the mouse.

• If you must use a mouse much of the time and you're still using an "old-fashioned" nonergonomic mouse, stop by a computer store and try out the new ergonomic ones, and also trackballs and touch pads. People are highly individual in their preferences. Find what works best for you, and either buy it for yourself or ask your employer to supply it.

• If you do more mousing than typing, put a clipboard on your lap and place the mouse there.

• Sit close to your desk so you don't have to reach for the mouse.

• If you must lean on your elbows, find foam pads to put under them to reduce pressure and avoid injury.

• Long fingernails are a hazard to typing hands. If you have to flatten your fingers to keep your nails out of the way, choose health over beauty and cut your nails just long enough to be seen when you hold up your hands with the palms facing you.

• If your chair doesn't provide support for the lumbar curve in your lower back, roll up a hand towel and place it there. A waist pack that is big enough to hold the rolled-up towel and buckled in front will keep the lumbar roll in place without your having to think about it. It may look funny if you wear it to the cafeteria, but your back will think you are beautiful.

• • • • • • • • • • • • • • • • •

Working Out at Work

You can exercise during your break to relieve the tension that comes from working in a fixed or awkward position. I suggest you try the following exercises, which have been adapted for people with fibromyalgia.[3] Do not do these exercises if you are already experiencing frequent pain in your back, neck, or shoulders or numbness and tingling in your hands and arms. If this is the case, see a doctor and do the exercises he or she prescribes for you. Exercises should be done slowly; focus on what you are doing, and feel your muscles as they move. This is a relaxation period, not a race. Do not stretch to the point of discomfort or pain. Exercise in flat shoes or your stockinged feet, not with your heels higher than the balls of your feet.

1. Standing or seated, keep your head facing forward and relax your shoulders. Shrug your shoulders up toward your ears. Hold them for a count of three. Relax. Repeat up to ten times, depending on how it feels.

2. Standing or seated, keep your head facing forward and your shoulders relaxed. Let your arms hang loosely at your sides. Slowly drop your chin to your chest. Hold for a count of three. Slowly raise your chin until it is tipped slightly toward the ceiling. Hold for a count of three. Slowly return to the starting position and repeat up to five times.

3. In the same position, turn your head to the right as far as you can comfortably. Do not raise or lower your chin.

Hold for a count of three, then return to the starting position. Turn your head to the left as far as you can without discomfort. Hold for a count of three. Slowly return to the starting position. Repeat up to five times.

4. In the same position, slowly drop your right ear toward your right shoulder, keeping your shoulder relaxed; do not raise it. Do not force your head to tilt. Hold for a count of three and return to the starting position. Now drop your left ear toward your left shoulder without forcing or pushing, and without raising your left shoulder. Count to three. Then return your head slowly to the starting position. Repeat up to five times.

5. Do this one seated. Put your left hand under your left buttock, keeping your left arm relaxed and slightly bent. Cradle the top of your head with your right hand. Gently pull your head downward toward your right knee as far as you can go comfortably. Do not strain. Keep your back upright; don't bend forward. The idea is to stretch your neck. Count to ten and return to the starting position. Now reverse sides, right hand under right buttock, left hand cradling your head and pulling toward your left knee. Count to ten and return to the starting position. Once is enough for this exercise.

6. Stand comfortably with your feet slightly apart in flat shoes or stockinged feet. Don't lock your knees. Keep your head balanced over your spine, looking straight ahead. Bend your elbows slightly, bringing your hands in front of your body and your elbows out to the sides. Move your elbows back and squeeze your shoulder blades closer together. Continue to face forward. Count to three and relax. Now round your shoulders forward while dropping your chin toward your chest, elbows still bent, and hands coming in front of your body. Count to three and relax. Return to the starting position. Do this exercise up to ten times.

7. Stand with your feet slightly apart and knees slightly bent. Bending at the hips, rest your hands lightly on your thighs and look at the floor. Slowly twist your body to the right, leading with your left shoulder. Keep looking down with your neck relaxed. Hold for a count of ten, then return to the starting position. Now twist to the left, leading with your right shoulder. Be aware of your head and neck, keeping them relaxed. Hold for a count of ten, then go back to the starting position. Do this exercise once only.

If you already have a cumulative trauma injury, use the information in this chapter to augment what you are already doing to treat it. If you have been ignoring pain and numbness that may signal a work-related injury, now is the time to start paying attention to it. If you have escaped injury so far and are determined to avoid any, you need to make a lifelong commitment to improving your posture and working conditions.

4

Going Places with Fibromyalgia

When I was diagnosed, I had the same ambivalent feelings that most people with FM have. I was devastated at the thought of having a chronic and incurable disorder, and relieved to have my suspicion validated that something was wrong and I wasn't just the victim of my own imagination. The sadness lasted for about forty-eight hours. During that time I could think of little more than all the wonderful experiences I'd had in my life that I could never repeat, and all the things I'd never done that were now impossible.

Then I realized that I was still the same person I was before the diagnosis. Anything I could do before I heard of fibromyalgia I could still do now. Anything I had intended to try I could still try. All that had changed was that I had a name for my problem. Since then I've made several cross-country trips without significant difficulty. Had I convinced myself that FM made me unable to travel, the quality of my life would now be poorer than it is.

In this chapter we'll look at getting around by air, automobile, and on foot. Traveling when you have fibromyalgia can be without distress if you plan well and take precautions as needed.

Airports and Airplanes

Big-city airports can be very stressful. From the moment you get onto the airport access road, cars whiz by. Signs with enormous amounts of information appear, and if you slow down to read them you run the risk of getting hit by a car six inches behind your rear bumper. Parking is usually far from the terminal, served by a shuttle bus onto which you must somehow load yourself and your luggage. Once inside the terminal there are more signs, people rushing everywhere, and loudspeaker announcements that might be made by people who couldn't care less whether anyone understands them.

The first rule of air travel is this: Your enjoyment of the trip decreases as the size of your luggage increases. In other words, pack as little as possible. I've learned to pack for a five-day trip using a suitcase that fits into the overhead compartment on the airplace and a carry-on bag that fits under the seat in front of me.

Days before I start packing I make lists. I plan what I will wear each day and add a pair of slacks and a sweater for evenings when I don't have to go anywhere. Unless I'm being met at my destination by someone for whom I have to look businesslike, I dress comfortably, not fashionably, for the flight. Loose slacks or a long skirt are what I choose. I have a suit that packs without wrinkling; that's usually my mainstay. Men on business trips wear the same suit day after day; why shouldn't I? Men don't pack extra shoes, and neither do I. The shoes I wear to travel are comfortable for walking, and that's all I need. I pack a pair of sweatpants, a T-shirt, and my sneakers for working out in the hotel's exercise room. I stuff the sneakers with socks, hose, and anything else that's small and compressible, to save space in the suitcase. Every item that I pack has to earn its way. I carry a small flashlight, a tiny sewing kit, and a few other items that are hard to find (or expensive) in a hotel. If I can possibly live for a few days without something, I don't pack it. If not having an item could ruin my trip or, at least, make me less able to accomplish what I've set out to do, I consider it worth packing.

My suitcase has wheels and a handle. My carry-on bag slides over the handle and sits on the top of the suitcase, so I have one hand free when I roll them. Nothing hangs off my shoulder. In the carry-on I carry my "bathroom," a case that holds my toiletry items, pillbox, and a leak-proof water bottle. I rarely check my suitcase, but if for some reason I must, I have with me the things I need most in case the suitcase is delayed or lost in transit. Instead of carrying a purse, I wear a waist pack to hold my wallet and plane ticket. The airlines don't count that as one of the two bags you're allowed to take on the airplane.

Some airports are so garishly lit that they can induce a headache, so I wear sunglasses. This may make me appear a bit eccentric, but if movie stars can do it, why can't I? One of the worst things about travel, for me, is the sensory overload. Sunglasses are one way to diminish that effect.

When I make my flight reservations, if I'm going to have to change planes, I ask the reservation agent about the distance between gates and the possibility of getting wheeled transportation if I need it. I'm not a small woman. I hate asking for a wheelchair, but if that's all that is available, I do so—and I tip the person who pushes me as generously as I can. Wherever possible, I ask to be met at the gate by an electric cart. Sturdy airline people younger than my children use them, so I don't think I'm taking the place of someone who is really disabled.

I have a folding cane that fits into my carry-on bag, and I use it if I am even slightly tired. I've had some fairly dramatic falls when I am overtired, and that's something I try to avoid. The cane comes in handy when it's time to board the plane. I'm one of those people who "need a little extra time," as the gate agents say, so I get up to board ahead of the crowd when they call for people with handicaps and those traveling with small children. Because I look healthy, some gate agents will challenge me if I try to board before the row on my ticket is called—but not if I'm carrying a cane. It's better that I board early, because I move more slowly than the average traveler. I think people would rather have me seated than have to stand in the aisle behind me while I settle myself in my seat.

I try to reserve an aisle or bulkhead seat on the plane. When I get to the airport, if I don't already have the bulkhead seat, I ask if it is available. It's much more comfortable for a long-legged person like me. Either way, I can get up and pace the aisle when the seat belt sign is off. I also do exercises such as flexing and relaxing my calf muscles and wiggling my toes. They help circulation and partially alleviate the pain of sitting. I always take one of those little airplane pillows and put it in the small of my back to provide lumbar support.

Because the climate in an airliner is drier than a desert, the risk of dehydration is significant. Among the symptoms of dehydration are fatigue, mental confusion, and headache. Dehydration also can cause muscle spasms. None of us with FM needs any more of these symptoms than we already have. When the complimentary drink cart comes around, I request mineral water or club soda. If you ask for the whole can rather than just a cup with lots of ice and little liquid, most flight attendants will comply. On flights of more than two hours, I'm not shy about asking for seltzer water every hour or so. I don't accept tap water from the airplane galley sink. That water can stay in a holding tank for days on end, a thought that doesn't appeal to me.

I rarely drink anything alcoholic, and I certainly wouldn't do so on an airplane. Both alcohol and coffee promote dehydration. For every six ounces of coffee you drink, you give back eight ounces of fluid. If you keep yourself well hydrated, your trip will be much more comfortable.

What to eat in flight poses an interesting question. Your goal should be to eat as normally as possible. If you're like most people with fibromyalgia, you need to pay attention to food intake to keep your blood sugar level stable. The risk of a reactive hypoglycemic episode is considerable, because it's often quite difficult to avoid refined sugar in an airline meal. Read the list of ingredients on the packet of salad dressing, for example, and you'll probably find that sugar is one of the first ingredients, which are listed in order of their presence in the product, largest amounts first.

Furthermore, airline meals have become quite unpredictable in recent years. Depending on the economic climate and what they think customers care about, airlines compete either for the lowest fares or the best service. When competition focuses on price, the "meal service" is likely to consist of a bag of peanuts or pretzels and a soft drink, or a sandwich at most. When service rules, you can expect a salad, entrée, vegetable, and dessert (which you'd be wise to skip). The only way to know what to expect is to ask the agent who books your flight. If a meal is to be served, you might want to ask if special meals are available for people with dietary restrictions. You're probably better off asking for a diabetic tray, although it's not unheard of for diabetic meals to include sugar. A vegetarian meal is probably safe. Asking for a sugar-free meal will probably not get you what you need. Food manufacturers put sugar into the most surprising things (read the label on a can of green beans next time you shop), and the people who prepare airline meals are unlikely to think of hidden sugar. Also, many sugar-free foods are sweetened with the sugar substitute aspartame, which for some of us is at least as bad as sugar. One possible solution is to pack your own food. I usually carry a bag of nuts or some trail mix, another product whose label you must read. Some trail mixes are high in refined sugar.

Time Zone Changes and Jet Lag

Even NDAs experience jet lag when they fly cross-country. If you fly from Boston to San Francisco, a distance of 2,700 miles, you arrive three hours earlier than your body clock's setting. As little as an hour's disruption of the sleep schedule can be difficult for people with fibromyalgia. Careful planning can reduce your discomfort.

By taking the following four steps, I was able to minimize the effects of jet lag on a trip to Britain. I'd recommend this strategy to anyone, but especially to people with fibromyalgia.

1. Counting the day of your trip as Day 5, begin on Day 1 to alternate days of low-calorie (about 900), high-complex-carbohydrate meals (mainly fruits and vegetables) and high-calorie (about 2,000), high-protein meals. The day of the trip should be a low-calorie day.

2. On the flight, pass up alcoholic drinks and drink lots of water. Sparkling water gets into your bloodstream faster than plain water does. Mineral water is better than tap water; all airlines carry both kinds of bottled water but will give them to you only if you ask. Don't let yourself become dehydrated.

3. When possible after arrival, get out into the daylight (sun, if you're lucky) without sunglasses for about three hours. Walk as much of that time as you can.

4. Follow the same routine on the way home, if possible.

Frequent travelers have a rule of thumb that says jet lag will last one day for each time zone you cross. By following this regimen, you can reduce that period considerably. If you can't follow the suggested diet before you head home, avoid alcohol and eat as sparingly as possible. The most important part of the routine is the walk in the sun, which you should do as soon as you can. It helps reset your internal clock.

Another possibility is to take melatonin, the hormone that tells your body when it's time to sleep, during the flight at the time you will want to go to sleep at the destination city the next night. You might even adjust your internal clock before you leave home by using melatonin for a few nights at the hour you will be going to sleep in the destination city. (For more about melatonin, see chapter 5, on sleep.) Or, if melatonin is not for you, try shifting your normal going-to-bed routine by fifteen minutes each night in the direction of bedtime at your destination.

For brief trips involving time zone changes of an hour or two, there is another alternative: Don't time-shift at all. If it doesn't interfere with your plans, you might simply observe the same routine while you're away that you do at home. You'll be a bit out of sync with those around you, but if it doesn't matter to you this might be the easiest way of all to travel. I've even done this on a trip from Eastern to Pacific time when my business required me to be on the West Coast for only two days. It was the easiest trip I've ever made.

Traveling by Car

If time doesn't matter, you might prefer to drive to your destination. Statistically, flying is safer, but I find driving less taxing. I can listen to music. I don't have to worry about changing flights, pushing luggage around for what seems like miles on end, or dealing with crowds of people. Automobile engine noise bothers me far less than the roar of an airplane's engines. I can drink water whenever I feel like it and set my own pace.

However, driving brings its own problems: The underlying tension of being in control of a car, the need to be alert to everything within sight, and the need to hold your arms in roughly the same position for long periods. However, some techniques can reduce the discomfort that comes from driving.

First, consider how you sit in the car. You can sit in a way that strains your back, shoulders, and arms, or you can adopt a posture that minimizes fatigue. Next time you drive, pay attention to how your body feels. Do you find it necessary to tip your head forward to see the road? If so, the angle of the seat may have caused you to lean back too far. An upright posture with your head balanced over your spine will probably ease strain on your neck. Do you have to hold your arms straight out to reach the steering wheel? Do you have to extend your leg fully to press on the brake or clutch? If either or both are true, the seat is probably pushed back too far. You should be able to use the pedals with your knees slightly bent. However, if your car is equipped with an air bag, you're safest if the compartment in which it is stored is at least ten inches away from your face and chest. Most of us learned in driver's ed to hold the steering wheel at the two and ten o'clock positions, but accepted practice today, particularly where air bags are installed, is more like five o'clock and seven o'clock. Not only does this keep your hands on the wheel if the air bag deploys, but it also allows you to hold your elbows close to your body in the position most often preferred by people who have fibromyalgia.

Lumbar support may make your driving experience much more pleasant. A hand towel rolled up into a cylinder makes a perfectly fine lumbar roll.

If you find it difficult to reach behind yourself to put on your seat belt, try taking hold of the shoulder portion as you get into the car. With practice you can seat yourself and fasten the buckle with a single motion.

Many people with fibromyalgia find themselves disoriented when they are driving, even in familiar places. I have a notebook in which I keep sticky notes on which I have written directions to places I go outside my normal errand-running destinations. I place the appropriate directions on the dashboard before I leave home. People who don't always have their rights and lefts sorted out can use arrows on their directions instead of the words. I've never been very good at reading maps, so my directions are always in words. If someone sends me a map to use for directions, I trace the route on the map and then write out the directions myself.

Disabled Parking

Some people think those who have fibromyalgia have no right to disabled parking. I disagree. If you had arthritis that caused as much pain on walking as many of us experience with fibromyalgia, you wouldn't hesitate for a moment to ask for the right to park close to your destination. Arthritis is a publicly accepted condition involving chronic pain; fibromyalgia has a way to go to be so universally accepted. Still, we know how much we hurt, and we have a right to relief just as an arthritic person does.

My position on disabled parking has changed over the years. For a long time, I was confused about whether I was entitled to it because my physical abilities are so variable. Sometimes I can walk without trouble, and other times fifty feet is too far for me. Also, while I can usually get out of the car and walk to the store entrance with no problem, by the time I'm finished shopping I'm apt to be staggering and in danger of falling. I hesitated for a long while before mentioning the subject of a disabled parking placard to my doctor, but she didn't hesitate for a moment before advising that I should have one.

Most states issue both placards, which you hang from the rearview mirror or place on the dashboard, and license plates. Generally, if you qualify for one, you qualify for both. I prefer a placard, because I can take it with me if I go in someone else's car. If the person to whom the placard is assigned is getting out of the car, the placard is valid no matter who owns the car or who is driving. Most states honor placards from another state. If you get a license plate, only the car to which it is attached has the right to park in a disabled spot.

The procedure involved in obtaining a placard or license plate differs from state to state. The department that issues driver's licenses and automobile number plates will tell you how to apply. In Massachusetts, where I live, you obtain the application form from the Registry of Motor Vehicles. Your doctor fills out the side that asks for medical information, and you fill out the side that asks for personal information: your name, address, driver's license number (if you have one; you don't have to be a driver to qualify for either placard or license plate), and date of birth. I had to include a passport photo with the application. The photo is laminated onto the placard, identifying me as the only legal user of the privilege.

On my application, the categories of disability included blindness, chronic lung disease, cardiovascular disease, arthritis, loss of the use of one or both feet or hands, and "other." In this last category, my doctor wrote, "Fibromyalgia." And for the requested description of functional disability, she added, "Severe fatigue and muscle pain with activity. Walking more than fifty feet can be extremely difficult."

The registry replied with a form letter asking that the physician clarify mobility limitations and say whether I use an ambulatory aid. This is what my doctor wrote:

> You have requested additional information on my patient, Miryam Williamson, regarding her fibromyalgia. Fibromyalgia is a chronic, incurable disease with permanent mobility limitations. Although the mobility limitations fluctuate at times, patients with fibromyalgia are chronically and permanently unable to walk significant distances without severe fatigue. In addition, she has major pain ambulating. She does use a cane as an ambulatory aid, particularly when her walking is extremely painful or when she is in danger of falling from fatigue.

That was all the registry needed to know. I now have a permanent placard clipped to the visor of my car. In the more than two years I've had it, I think I've used it about a dozen times, but I don't know what I would have done without it when I needed it.

If you're the passenger and riding strains your neck, you may want to consider bringing a cervical collar with you and wearing it half the time you are in the car. Most physical therapists don't recommend using a cervical collar unless it is absolutely necessary, on the theory that relying on its support will weaken neck muscles. However, wearing it for half-hour intervals won't hurt, and you may find it restful.

If the trip will take more than an hour and you must arrive at a specific time, leave home ten minutes earlier for every hour you expect to be driving. Use those ten minutes for a rest break. Get out of the car, do a bit of stretching, and walk around a bit to maintain mental clarity and reduce stiffness.

Visiting

Whether the place you will stay is a hotel or the home of someone in your circle of family and friends, you'll be sleeping in a strange bed, eating strange food, and living according to an unfamiliar schedule.

If your destination is a hotel, you'll want to make reservations in advance to avoid the inconvenience of finding it full, as can happen if a conference or convention is scheduled for the same time as your trip. Take the opportunity to ask about facilities and make your needs known. If your normal regimen includes an exercise program, you'll be better off if you choose a hotel that has fitness facilities. People accustomed to a daily walk often find themselves in trouble when they register at a hotel situated where walking outside is impossible, a common situation in many parts of the United States. You'll be much better able to withstand the rigors of travel if you maintain your exercise schedule. Having a treadmill or stationary bike available may make the difference between a pleasant trip and one that makes you ill.

Ask for a room on a nonsmoking floor (unless you're a smoker, of course) that is not too far from the elevator but not next to it, either. People sometimes congregate near the elevators and may not be aware that their conversations can disturb other guests. Consider taking earplugs and eyeshades with you to minimize noise and light in your room. Protect yourself as much as you can from things that can disturb your sleep.

Think carefully about the items you need at home to be able to function at your highest level, and try to supply those items when you are away from home. For me, the major issue is drinking water. Chlorine, which is added to public water supplies everywhere in the United States, upsets my digestive system, so I can't drink tap water in my hotel room or even in a restaurant. I pack a quart or two of water from home when I travel, and buy bottled springwater as soon as possible after I check into the hotel, which usually means finding a nearby supermarket or large pharmacy. It's not a perfect solution, but at least I avoid the chlorine. If all else fails, I buy water from the hotel gift shop, but there the bottles are apt to be smaller and the prices outrageous.

Most people who have fibromyalgia need to go to the bathroom during the night. Having a small flashlight to help you find your way without turning on lights can make the difference between getting back to sleep and staying awake the rest of the night. Melatonin is secreted mostly in the dark. People vary greatly in the way their secretion of melatonin reacts to light. In some, as little as five minutes' exposure to light can halt melatonin's production, waking them completely. This effect may be triggered in even less time; studies of shorter durations of light exposure have yet to be published.[4]

If you're traveling by car, consider taking your own pillows. Otherwise, when you get to your room don't be shy about calling the housekeeping department and asking for extra pillows.

Most hotel rooms have controls for the air-conditioning and heating systems, but they are not always easy to find. If you need to be shown how to adjust the room temperature and ventilation, call the front desk from your room and ask for help. Let the hotel staff know what you need in order to be comfortable. Your comfort is (or should be) their primary concern, and they can't know what you need unless you tell them.

Familiarize yourself with the room service menu and determine whether having a meal delivered to your room involves added costs. Some hotels add a room service charge to their restaurant prices, and some do not. Sometimes, when you're tired, it's worth the extra money to eat in your room, but it's better to know about this surcharge before you place your order rather than be presented with a bill you weren't prepared for.

Staying with family or friends can be a bit trickier, unless your host understands fibromyalgia and is sensitive to your needs. Think hard about visiting people who think FM is a kind of hypochondria. Even in the most supportive environments, guest room beds are often less than ideal, and your host may not be aware of your special sleep needs. Try to find out, as delicately and politely as you can, what the bed is like and how dark and quiet the room will be. Just as with a hotel, earplugs and eyeshades may come in handy. Unfortunately, many people find it impossible to sleep well the first night in a strange bed. Don't plan a lot of activities for your first full day away from home; bear in mind that you may not be at your best then.

Talk frankly with your host before you arrive about any special dietary needs you may have. People who don't live with allergies often don't think to ask their guests about this. The person who has invited you probably wants you to be comfortable while you visit. If you fail to be open about your needs, you're not doing anyone any favors.

At the same time, you'll surely want to reduce the inconvenience your visit causes your hosts. Do what you can to help, and don't beat yourself up over what you can't do. With careful planning, your travels can be a pleasure. Unfortunately, for people with fibromyalgia, the spontaneous "just pick up and go" trip is rarely a success.

Walking

Life isn't much fun if you can't go anywhere, and going places usually involves some amount of walking. For most of my life I could neither walk nor stand for long without significant pain. Now I can do both—most of the time. Being able to stand at social gatherings and walk when I need to has improved the quality of my life enormously.

The trick that helps me most with both walking and standing is one I learned from a teacher of the Alexander Technique (more about this in chapter 9). She taught me to carry myself regally, pulling myself up to my full height and especially trying to increase the distance between my pelvis and rib cage. Now, when I feel that familiar pain in my hip, I pretend I am a queen appearing before her subjects. The relief from pain is instantaneous, and the more I do this, the more habitual proper carriage becomes.

I don't see how I'll ever get over my tendency to fall when I am tired. I've had all the tests and examinations required to rule out any specific cause, but the problem persists. The sensation, when it happens, is like stepping into a hole. I put my foot down, but my leg just doesn't catch my weight. It's as if there's no leg there. My solution is to use a cane when I'm apt to get tired. Used properly, a cane can also help reduce fatigue.

If you choose to use a cane, its height should be such that your arm is slightly bent when you hold it by your side. The top of the curve in the cane's handle should be about on a level with your hip joint when you are standing. Some metal canes are easily adjustable. You can remove the rubber tip from a wooden cane and shorten it with a hacksaw. Most medical supply stores will make the adjustment for you if you ask. If holding a cane makes your hand hurt, buy a length of foam pipe insulation from the hardware store and slide it over the handle of the cane.

Experts differ on whether you should hold the cane on your weaker or stronger side. If you can see a physical therapist for a lesson in using the cane, that's ideal. If not, try it yourself and you'll probably know soon enough which position and technique work for you. I hold my cane on my right side next to the leg that sometimes forgets it's a leg, and the cane and leg move together. As I step forward with my right leg, I swing the cane forward, too. That way, if my leg doesn't do its job, the cane is there to support me. People with hip pain generally find it works better to put the cane on the side opposite to the sore hip and synchronize the cane and the leg on the sore side so that they always have a three-point support.

Whatever you do, don't get into the habit of leaning on your cane. It's there as an aid; if you put much weight on it, you'll have a sore hand and shoulder in no time. If you use your cane properly, you'll probably walk as though you don't need one. That's the whole idea.

If your pain is in both legs, you may be better off with forearm crutches. Their drawback is that they occupy both your hands, so you need a backpack or waist pack to carry things in.

My cane folds to about a foot in length. I normally keep it in my handbag or briefcase and use it only when I feel I need it. It's not that I'm afraid of becoming dependent on it, but that when I don't need it it's more trouble than it's worth.

When you climb stairs, lead with the good leg going up, the bad leg going down. Hold on to the handrail. If your knee bothers you, try to avoid bearing weight on it when it is bent. This means putting both feet on each step, baby style, but the benefit to your knee makes it worthwhile.

The right pair of shoes can make a world of difference in your ability to walk. You don't necessarily need the latest in high-technology walking shoes. In fact, the right pair of shoes may be in your closet (or on your feet) right now. If your feet, legs, hips, and/or lower back hurt when you walk for more than a few minutes, take inventory of your shoe collection and decide whether a new pair is worth the cost.

Take your shoes out of the closet and line them up in front of you. Set aside any shoes that have heels more than an inch and a half high. High heels strain your knees and back and also your feet. Save them for going to sit-down events such as movies or concerts. If you wear high heels to parties where people mostly stand around, you'll wind up sitting and miss most of the fun, or standing in pain while still missing most of the fun. If you're accustomed to wearing high heels, however, don't choose a perfectly flat shoe for walking. You'll strain your Achilles tendon, that tough cablelike sinew that runs from the bottom of your calf to the top of your heel. Instead, plan to stretch that tendon gradually by wearing increasingly lower heels.

Look at the heels and soles of your most-used shoes. Are they worn down evenly, or do you see signs of a faulty gait, such as heels that slope toward the inside or outside of the shoe? Do both shoes reflect the same amount of use, or is one heel or sole thinner than the other? If the bottoms of these shoes reflect uneven use, take yourself and them to a podiatrist (a foot doctor), orthopedist, physical therapist, or other expert in posture and gait for corrective exercises. Perhaps shoe inserts would help you stand and walk with even pressure on all parts of your feet.

Assuming the bottoms of your shoes are wearing out evenly, you can continue searching your shoe collection for an appropriate pair for walking. Look again at the soles, but this time look at what they are made of. Leather soles are acceptable for standing and short walks, but for serious walking you need rubber or composition soles that provide maximum shock absorption. Put back in the closet any shoes that have leather soles. Flex the remaining shoes and reject those that bend anywhere other than where your foot bends, at the ball.

The heels of walking shoes should be as wide as the shoe itself and should also have shock-absorbing capabilities. Put back in the closet shoes with narrow, leather, or wooden heels and those that have metal plates nailed on to lengthen the life of the heels. Not only do these increase the stress to your feet and legs, but the metal "taps" also mask effects of an improper gait and delay any corrective action on your part.

The heel counter is the back of the shoe itself. It must be firm to keep your foot straight. Squeeze it from the top, sides, and back. If it yields too much to your pressure, the shoe will not give you the support you need. Remove from consideration as your primary walking shoe those with flexible counters. Reject, too, any shoes whose heel counters are loose enough to let your heel slide up and down as you walk. The resulting friction is likely to lead to blisters.

Look at the insole and arch of the shoes you are still considering. A cushioned sole is best, or, if the shoe has enough room, you can buy a cushioned insert at the drugstore. If you have high arches, you may benefit from shoes that have built-in arch supports or from a purchased insole that includes an arch support.

The best uppers are those made of soft, but not mushy, leather. Cloth is acceptable, too, if it is neither too stiff nor too soft. Reject shoes whose uppers are made of synthetic materials. They won't adapt to the unique shape of your feet, and they will prevent your feet from breathing, trapping moisture and providing a friendly environment for athlete's foot and other fungal infections. Wet feet are also prone to developing blisters. Laces, buckles, and Velcro-type fasteners are fine. Slip-ons and loafers are acceptable if the shoes fit properly and are made of material that won't stretch and become too loose.

If you have any pointy-toe shoes left in the pile you are considering, put them aside now. Your toes need room to wiggle. If the toe box is too tight, your toes will be pressed together, possibly causing corns and bunions. Watch out, too, for shoes that are too narrow, particularly those that compress your smallest toe. Most women wear shoes that are too narrow for them.

If you've run out of shoes to consider for serious walking, it's time to go shoe shopping. Before you go, though, trace the outline of both bare feet on paper and bring the tracing to the store with you. The tracing should be made when you have been up and walking for a while. Ideally you'll be standing when you trace; it may be easier to stand up straight and ask someone else to trace your feet for you. At the shoe store your tracing should match or fit just inside the sole of the shoes you are considering.

Always shop for shoes in the afternoon or evening. Everyone's feet swell during the day, even if they don't have FM. Try on shoes with the same kind and weight of socks you expect to wear with them. Besides using the outline of your foot to rule out shoes not worth trying on, ask to have your feet measured. Don't accept the salesperson's assertion that shoes that feel a bit too tight will stretch with wearing. Good, properly fitted shoes don't need to be broken in.

Some people routinely buy their shoes a half-size longer and one size wider than the measuring tool specifies. This may be a good idea, or it may lead to blisters if the shoes are really too big, not just a bit loose. Another way to buy shoes for people who hate to go shopping or who want a trial period in which to wear them is by mail order from a company that allows returns of shoes that have been worn. Two companies with this policy are Massey's and Footprints. (Their addresses are in the "Resources" section of this book.) If you make a mistake, Massey's will accept returns for up to thirty days and Footprints for six months. You pay the shipping both ways, but you won't have to argue to get a refund.

5

To Sleep, Perchance to Dream

Nearly everyone with fibromyalgia has trouble sleeping. Estimates of sleep dysfunction in people with FM range from 75 to 99 percent. Some people with fibromyalgia think they are sleeping if they are unaware of the time's passage during the night, although they awaken tired and sore. Some physicians, uninformed about the special relationship between fibromyalgia and sleep, consider their patients' complaints of poor sleep as trivial. Both situations are unfortunate. If you can achieve sleep that is restful and restorative, you will have made great progress toward getting the rest of your fibromyalgia symptoms under control. If you are not waking up rested and refreshed, your sleep needs attention and repair.

In studies by Harvey Moldofsky, M.D., and others, apparently healthy people developed symptoms of FM, particularly muscle pain, digestive upsets, and cognitive problems, when they were deprived of restful sleep for three consecutive nights. To accomplish this, Moldofsky hooked up the study subjects to electroencephalographic (EEG) machines, which measure brain wave activity. When the machines registered deep sleep, an alarm sounded and the subjects were awakened, then allowed to go back to sleep. (This scenario may sound dreadfully familiar to those of us with fibromyalgia, except that we tend to bob up to shallow sleep spontaneously, without any help from an alarm.) Once they were allowed to sleep normally, the subjects' symptoms disappeared. Significantly, athletes in the study group recovered more rapidly than the others did.

Sleep scientists generally recognize two kinds of problems: difficulty in getting to sleep; and waking too often or too early, unable to get back to sleep. Many people have both problems. In discussions with your doctor, it helps to be specific about the sleep patterns you are experiencing.

Fibromyalgia adds a third dimension, a kind of sleep in which the sleeper remains semialert. Most people with fibromyalgia spend their nights in a state of perpetual wakefulness, with rapid alpha brain waves intruding into slow-wave delta sleep. In adults, about 80 percent of the growth hormone secreted by the pituitary gland is produced during deep sleep. People with fibromyalgia are usually deficient in growth hormone, which is responsible for much of the body's repair work. Therefore, it's no surprise that people who don't get delta sleep start the day feeling sore and achy, as though they've had a run-in with a truck. Insomnia and the resulting deficiency in growth hormone may also be responsible for some obesity found in many people with fibromyalgia. Growth hormone moves nutrients in the bloodstream into muscle and away from fat.

Sleep is important for other reasons, too. Disturbed sleep is associated with cognitive dysfunction—poor memory and the inability to think clearly. Poor sleep disrupts the immune system. One theory says that insomnia causes increased production of certain immune system chemicals called cytokines. These are known to have strong effects on the brain, causing fatigue and cognitive problems in illnesses including influenza and in autoimmune diseases such as multiple sclerosis and lupus. Fibromyalgia is not an autoimmune disease, but it is associated with heightened immune system activity. Cytokines increase general body aches. These same cytokines are also used in some chemotherapy treatments to combat cancer by stimulating the body's own defense system. Cytokines used in chemotherapy make patients feel particularly awful. The cytokines produced to fight the flu virus are what make you feel so achy and tired when you have it. It's no accident that people describe FM's muscle aches as feeling like a bad case of flu.

Sleep Disrupters

Alpha-wave intrusion into delta sleep is only one cause of sleep disturbance in people with fibromyalgia. Obstructive sleep apnea (OSA) is common, particularly in men. According to one estimate, nearly half of all men with FM have OSA.[5] It's not as common among women. OSA is a mechanical problem. During sleep the soft part of the back of the throat relaxes so fully that it blocks the airway. The sleeper stops breathing momentarily, then takes in air with a sharp gasp that disturbs his or her sleep. In some people this can happen 100 or more times a night. OSA can usually be treated successfully by a neurologist who specializes in sleep disturbances. (A similar but unrelated condition called central sleep apnea, so named because it arises in the central nervous system, can be life-threatening and demands medical intervention.)

OSA is easy to spot if you sleep with someone. If you sleep alone and think you may have this problem, your health care practitioner can help you decide whether you should have a sleep study done. Generally, a sleep study is conducted at a hospital. You will probably be encouraged to bring your own pillow and take any medications you normally take. You will go to bed in your own nightclothes, be hooked up to an EEG machine, and be monitored during the night. A couple of apneas per hour is not unusual, but if enough occur to disturb your sleep the doctor will probably prescribe a CPAP (continuous positive airway pressure) machine. This device pumps air into your nose through a mask. Some people report it takes a few nights to get used to sleeping this way, but the success rate for people with OSA who use these machines is high.

Nocturnal myoclonus, also known as periodic limb movements of sleep (PLMS), is a disturbance that can often be relieved with medication, usually a small dose of an anticonvulsive drug. Probably everyone has had the experience of an arm or leg jerking suddenly while falling asleep. This is normal, caused by a stray electrical discharge in the brain, and nothing to worry about. However, when those jerks continue during the night, they wake you continuously, making restful sleep impossible. As with OSA, if you sleep alone a sleep study may be the only way to ascertain whether you have this problem. Fixing it may be all it takes to get you restorative sleep and some relief from your FM symptoms.

Bruxism, the grinding of teeth during sleep, can cause both insomnia and pain in the temporomandibular joint, the jaw's hinge. Bruxism is most commonly thought to be caused by psychological stress, but a malocclusion of the jaw (or bad bite) can also cause it. A dentist skilled in treating jaw joint problems can make you a bite plate to be worn at night. This prevents, or at least reduces, the grinding.

Another possible cause of FM's sleep disturbance is an abnormal pattern of cortisol release, known as sleep-phase syndrome disorder. (See the Introduction for more information on cortisol.) People with this problem sleep well and for a normal amount of time, but not at the time of day when most people do. Allowed to sleep according to their own needs, such people can function well. Of course, sleep-phase disorder seriously disrupts normal life if one has a family and daytime responsibilities. If this sounds like you, don't take any drugs before reading the section on sleep hygiene that comes later in this chapter; the suggestions there may help you resolve the problem.

Fixing your sleep is not a cure for fibromyalgia, but it is an important component in improving the quality of your life. Once you are sleeping well and reliably most nights (the person who never experiences a night of insomnia is rare), your pain and other symptoms will almost certainly diminish.

• • • • • • • Snoring • • • • • • •

Snoring is a common problem among people with fibromyalgia—not their own snoring, but that of the person with whom they sleep. About one person in four snores habitually, so if you sleep with someone who snores, you have lots of company. Snoring is the subject of many stand-up comedy acts, but there's nothing funny about lying awake while the person next to you is loudly proclaiming how deeply he or she is sleeping. Not only is someone else's snoring harmful to a person who has fibromyalgia, but it can also poison a cherished relationship. It is in your best interest, the interest of your partner, and the health of the bond between you to take action.

• Try industrial-strength earplugs, the kind that people who operate noisy machinery use. They come in various sizes and have a series of flexible rings around a shaft that act as baffles to block noise. After you insert them, pull them out just a bit to flatten the rings against the ear canal. If they fit properly, you won't be aware that they are in place, but they'll block out all but the loudest snores.

• Try using a sound-conditioning machine to drown out the noise. Sound-conditioning machines may emit only "white noise," a soft signal that blots out other noises, or they may have settings to imitate rain, ocean sounds, or other sounds that induce relaxation. Stores that sell radios and electronic devices often stock such items.

• Find a peaceful time to start a discussion of the problem. Don't expect to solve it immediately, but do expect to solve it. Be careful not to sound hostile. Knowing your snoring is disturbing someone you care about must be terrible if you don't know how to stop it. Look for solutions rather than placing blame.

• Remember that alcoholic drinks and fatty foods increase the likelihood of snoring.

• Ask if it is all right to touch or push the snorer when the noise gets too loud. Some people become badly startled if they are touched when sleeping, and may react rather vigorously. People who do this usually know they do; it's up to you to ask.

• Ask the snorer to try an antisnoring aid. You can buy adhesive patches that widen the nostril openings, U-shaped devices that press on the nasal septum (the wall between the nostrils), and pillows with low ridges and a depression for the neck that holds the person's head straight. One or more of these may solve the problem.

• If the snorer has allergies or sinus problems, ask her or him to consider taking an antihistamine or decongestant before bed.

• Check the humidity in the bedroom. A room that is too dry makes snoring worse. Consider using a humidifier or vaporizer.

• Look into research in the use of radio-frequency energy to reduce heavy snoring and treat OSA, conducted in 1997 by the Stanford Sleep Disorders and Research Center, Stanford University, California. A device made by Somnus Medical Technologies was approved by the U.S. Food and Drug Administration in late 1997. Ask a sleep specialist.

• • • • • • • • • • • • • • • • • • •

Preparations That Promote Sleep

If you are currently feeling desperate about your inability to get restful sleep, you may be better off asking your health care professional for some medication to take for a while so you can get some rest. No sleep medicine should be taken for very long. One or two weeks is usually the limit of its effectiveness and safety. After a couple of weeks your liver gets more proficient at clearing the drug from your bloodstream, and you need more of the drug to get the desired effect. Still, if you're getting into bed at night knowing that you won't be able to sleep, a sleeping pill initially may help you get over that expectation, which will help with the rest of the steps you may take to solve your sleeping problem.

Some sleeping pills actually interfere with delta-level sleep. Before you take a medication prescribed by your physician, make sure that it won't do this. The preferred sleeping pill among people with fibromyalgia is zolpidem tartrate. Its brand name is Ambien. It is reported not to interfere with deep sleep.

One over-the-counter medication that some people find helpful is diphenhydramine, best known by its brand name, Benadryl. It is an antihistamine, used most often by people with allergies. However, some doctors recommend a 25 mg tablet before bedtime for sleep. If you want to try it, you should ask the pharmacist to let you see a package insert, which details precautions, conditions under which it should not be taken, and possible side effects. (Remember that no drug is without possible side effects. To decide on any new drug, you should weigh the risk of possible side effects against the benefit you hope to obtain.) Be sure to select a package of diphenhydramine that is for allergies and not also for colds and sinus problems. The multipurpose preparation contains a decongestant that is also a stimulant—not what you need for a good night's sleep.

Two less well known substances that some people with fibromyalgia find beneficial are the essential amino acid L-tryptophan and a related compound, 5-hydroxytryptophan (5-HTP).

Many people with fibromyalgia and other sleep disorders treated themselves with L-tryptophan in the 1980s, when it was available at low cost in health food stores. Then a batch contaminated during the manufacturing process was brought into the United States by the Japanese manufacturer Showa Denko, causing a painful and in a few cases deadly condition called eosinophilia myalgia syndrome (EMS).

The FDA wisely recalled L-tryptophan. (Later, it recalled Tylenol when contaminated capsules killed several people.) However, after it was determined that the cause of death was faulty manufacturing and not the amino acid L-tryptophan, the FDA refused to return L-tryptophan to the marketplace. (By contrast, Tylenol was allowed back on the shelves promptly after the source of contamination was determined.)

A 1995 article in the *Journal of Musculoskeletal Pain* questions the association of EMS with L-tryptophan, showing that some patients with the EMS diagnosis already had fibromyalgia and were no more disabled three years after the onset of EMS than they were before taking L-tryptophan.[6] On February 9, 1993, the U.S. patent office issued a patent for the use of L-tryptophan to treat and cure EMS, the very same condition that prompted the FDA to take L-tryptophan off the market in 1989.[7] Since L-tryptophan has never been banned for use in feeding formulas for two of the most vulnerable segments of the human race—infants and people fed by stomach tube because they are unable to take nourishment by mouth—one questions the claims that it is a danger to the public.

Today it is available from compounding pharmacies (pharmacies that can mix prescribed ingredients to make remedies not manufactured by pharmaceutical companies) at a cost roughly ten times its price before the FDA banned it, about the same cost as Prozac, which came on the market just before tryptophan was banned. Both L-tryptophan and Prozac increase the availability of serotonin, although they do so in different ways. Many people who are deficient in serotonin can benefit from either the amino acid L-tryptophan or the drug Prozac; therefore, the two products are competitors. If you want scientific evidence of the usefulness of L-tryptophan in treating insomnia, uncontaminated by the politics involved in its competition with Prozac, ask a medical librarian to help you find pertinent journal articles.[8]

Also available at compounding pharmacies is 5-HTP, the breakdown product of tryptophan. Both work by helping the body create serotonin, a brain chemical closely related to sleep. People with fibromyalgia have been found deficient in serotonin. Chemical depression also is often associated with low levels of serotonin. I have been taking 5-HTP since May 1995. It almost always helps me achieve good, restful sleep, and most of the time my pain level is no longer worth complaining about. Sources of L-tryptophan and 5-HTP are listed in the "Resources" section. Like everything else relating to fibromyalgia, they don't work for everyone, but many people have found one or the other quite beneficial. You may find them worth considering and discussing with your health care provider.

Another hormone some people find useful for sleep is melatonin. Secreted by the pineal gland, melatonin sets the body's clock, telling it when it is time to sleep. Unlike L-tryptophan, melatonin is sold in drugstores and health food stores in the United States. Melatonin can interfere with ovulation (indeed, it has widespread use as a birth control pill) and should not be used by anyone contemplating pregnancy. People with severe allergies, autoimmune diseases, and immune system cancers such as lymphoma and leukemia should not take it, either. An interesting thing about melatonin is that smaller doses are usually more effective than larger doses. For most people, doses of 1 mg or less are best.

Some herbs are credited with helping induce restorative sleep. Most often named are chamomile (a member of the goldenrod family, to be avoided by people with hay fever), valerian, skullcap, passionflower, vervain, and kava kava. Some of these are available in capsule form, others in bulk at the health food store. Herb teas are prepared by placing the loose herbs in water that is very hot, just short of simmering, and letting them steep until the tea is strong. If you wake up during the night and have trouble getting back to sleep, you might try drinking half a cup at bedtime and putting the cup by your bed to sip from later.

Don't make the mistake of thinking that because herbs are plants they are without possible side effects. Think of herbs as another kind of medicine, and do the same research on them that you'd do before taking a new drug.

You might also want to experiment with the aroma of lavender. A 1996 British study turned up evidence that the scent of lavender may be as effective as sleeping pills for some people. In a six-week trial, more than 100 nursing home residents had their hours of sleep measured for the first two weeks using tranquilizers, then for two weeks with no pills. Finally, experimenters diffused lavender oil into the patients' rooms. Sleep levels fell significantly during the middle two weeks, but patients reported their sleep was more restful with lavender.[9]

Sleep Hygiene

The place where you sleep should be as comfortable and nurturing as you can possibly make it. While you want your body to be warm when you sleep, the room you sleep in should be cool, well ventilated, and not too dry. You need a quiet place (or earplugs), one that is dark (or you can wear eyeshades), and a bed that works well for you. Firm mattresses are good for the spine but may put pressure on FM tender points and make some sleeping positions impossible. The ideal is a firm mattress with a soft pad on top. Some people like egg-crate foam pads. My choice is a feather bed, since I'm not allergic to feathers. For those who are but want this kind of softness, there are feather bed–like pads made of hypoallergenic materials. (See the "Resources" section for the names of some companies that specialize in products for people with allergies.)

Even more than mattresses, pillows are a matter of personal taste. Your pillow should support your neck, not just your head, for maximum restfulness. To find the right pillow thickness for you, stand with your shoulders and head touching a wall. Have someone measure the distance from the wall to the back of your neck. That's how thick your pillow should be when you compress it. You can also use a neck roll, tucked into your pillowcase, for support. Some people say that buckwheat pillows are a dream. Be careful if you buy one, though. Some are chemically treated, and their odor can make environmentally sensitive people quite uncomfortable. Smell before you buy, whatever the pillow you choose.

One of the hardest things for me to accept about FM is the need to be scrupulous about my sleep habits. I've always loved staying up late, even when raising a family prevented me from making up lost nighttime sleep in the morning. When my children were little, staying up late was the only way I could get time for myself. It wasn't until I was diagnosed and learned of the relationship between fibromyalgia and sleep that I realized my daytime well-being depended heavily on my nighttime routine.

There is simply no way around it: To feel your personal best—to have the best quality of life possible—you've got to get adequate sleep. Whether or not you are taking something to help you sleep, you have no choice about the basic rule of good sleep hygiene: You must go to bed and get up at the same time every day. This is especially true when you are embarking on a program to solve your sleep problems. The day may come when you can make an occasional exception, but not until you are confident of your ability to sleep. This may take months to achieve.

Some people do well on six hours of good sleep. Others need ten hours. If you remember a time when you slept well and can remember how much sleep you required then, let that number of hours be your initial target. If you've never slept well, choose eight hours, the average requirement for adults, as your goal. In either case, you may want to adjust your desired number of hours of sleep as you gain experience in working on this problem.

Count back from the time you want to (or must) wake up to

find the time you want to go to sleep. Start your going-to-bed routine an hour before that. Your presleep hour must be a time of winding down.

• • • Your Presleep Routine • • •

• Turn off the television, unless you can find something to watch that is pleasant. Cop shows, thrillers, and the news are bad bets. They're too stimulating.

• In cold weather, turn up the heat in your bedroom, or put an electric heating pad or hot-water bottle under the covers where the sorest part of your body will rest. (Turn down the heat and remove the heating pad or hot-water bottle before you get into bed.)

• Dim the lights; you want to see clearly, but you don't want bright light.

• Put on the kind of music that you find relaxing.

• Have a small snack—nothing sugary or fatty. Fruit or unsweetened fruit juice, a couple of crackers, or a banana and glass of milk are ideal. The banana and milk especially will increase the tryptophan available when you want to fall asleep.

• Avoid alcohol both at dinner and in the evening. Alcohol interferes with deep sleep. People who drink themselves to sleep feel worse in the morning, not better. If you're taking a sleeping pill, alcohol can increase its effect to the point where it stops your breathing. Never mix alcohol and sleeping drugs. If you're currently using alcohol or a mix of alcohol and pills as a sleep aid, please stop. Get help if you need it. Asking for help in such a situation is a sign of strength, not weakness.

• Time the taking of sleep aids, if any, to the time you want to be asleep. Zolpidem tartrate (Ambien) works fast and should be taken just before you get into bed. Some people find that amitriptyline (Elavil) is most effective if taken two or three hours before bedtime. You may need to experiment to find the best interval between taking sleep medication and getting into bed.

• Draw a warm bath, get into the tub, and soak for ten to twenty minutes, adding hot water if the bath starts to get cool. Roll a towel to make a pillow for your head. Try to submerge yourself up to your neck. Wash or just soak, but don't scrub.

• Get out of the tub, pat yourself dry, and put on your nightclothes (or don't, if you prefer).

• Try lavender—on your body, or in a pillow, candle, or oil diffuser.

● ● ● ● ● ● ● ● ● ● ● ● ● ● ● ● ●

When you do get into bed, turn out the light and smile. Smile? Yes, I mean it. I learned this technique from a woman with FM who uses humor to make herself feel better. I was skeptical at first, but trying it myself has convinced me that I feel better when I smile, even if I can't think of anything to smile about.

Smiling when you get into bed has another benefit. Take a moment to notice the muscles in your face right now. If you're not already smiling, they are probably tight. Now smile. Can you feel your whole face loosen up? That's the effect you're after—nice, loose muscles all over will help you fall asleep. One of my favorite going-to-sleep exercises is to raise my eyebrows once or twice, and then concentrate on making the muscles I just used as soft as possible. If the muscles of your face soften, particularly those in your forehead, the rest of your body will soften in response.

Don't Just Lie There

It's hard to smile when you get into bed expecting insomnia. You've got to give sleep a chance. Talk to yourself. Tell yourself you are going to learn to sleep well, and be patient with yourself while you learn. Don't actually try to sleep at first. Just make yourself as comfortable as you can, let your muscles go loose, and let your mind run free. If you find yourself thinking about something unpleasant, tell yourself, "No, I'm not going to think about that now," and turn your thoughts elsewhere. Think of something pleasant—a time when you had fun or were happy; a vacation, a party, a walk in the woods. If you're good at making pictures in your mind, be an artist. Paint a beautiful mental landscape, with trees, flowers, birds, animals. Let a gentle snowfall start, but with the sun still shining. Enjoy the sparkling of the snowflakes in the sun. You can think of anything you want to while you're resting in bed, provided it's not negative and worrisome.

Some people who write about insomnia say that if you are not asleep within fifteen or twenty minutes you should get out of bed and read or watch television until you get sleepy. This is not good advice for most people with FM. We may have experienced dysfunctional sleep for so long that we no longer get sleepy. Even now, I expect to lie in the dark for forty-five minutes to an hour after lights out, and I don't mind that. I use the time to think and to play with my imagination. It's my private time—nothing to do, no responsibilities, a time to explore my hopes and dreams.

Maybe sleep won't come for the first few nights, but you'll be no worse off than you were before you tried this technique. Stick with it. Don't give up. You're training your body and mind to get ready for sleep. They'll learn, if you're consistent in your efforts. If you are using prescription drugs for sleep, as time goes by, you may find you need less chemical assistance, but it may take months or even years. After three years of taking 5-HTP—which isn't strong enough to work unless I work with it, by the way—a few times recently I have forgotten to take it. I still slept, although not as well. When I finish writing this book, I'm going to try cutting down my dose a bit to see if I still need as much as I did when I started.

While you are lying there resting, if you start feeling that you simply must move your legs, a common experience for many people, do a flutter kick as though you were swimming for a minute or so. You're probably experiencing restless leg syndrome (different from nocturnal myoclonus), one of those things about which little is known. Giving your legs more activity than they bargained for often helps.

As you lie there resting your body and mind, you may find yourself starting to worry about things over which you have no control. There is a time during the presleep period when the protective shell within which we live during the day—the sleep specialist who told me about this called it *euthymia*, literally meaning "good mood"—peels away and we are without our normal defenses. If you can't turn your mind away from unpleasant thoughts, get up. Bed is no place for worrying. Take a drink of milk or juice, go to the bathroom, walk around the house a bit, and then climb back into bed and start over. If you do get up, though, don't turn on the lights. Leave a dim light burning in the hall or bathroom if you need it for safety, but don't let yourself face bright light until morning.

The reason for this is found in one word: *melatonin*, the hormone secreted by your pineal gland that tells your body it's time for sleep. Melatonin is produced in the dark. If you turn on the lights, you risk shutting it off. Don't take that chance.

Melatonin is the main reason sleep experts tell you not to read in bed. If it's light enough to read, it's too light to secrete melatonin. To be honest, I break that rule every night. Part of my relaxation routine involves reading a short story—rarely more than one and often not a whole one—before I turn out the light. I don't read novels, because I want a definite place to stop and don't want to get myself into a position where I have to keep turning pages to see how the situation resolves itself. I don't read nonfiction, because I think I have to be responsible for remembering what I've read. Reading for enjoyment is an important factor in the quality of my life, and the only time I get to do this is at the end of the day. If reading for pleasure is important to you, too, you can probably break the no-reading-in-bed rule as I do, if you're careful in your choice of reading material.

Wakening Too Often or Too Early

Some people have almost no trouble falling asleep but find they can't *stay* asleep. They sleep soundly for a couple of hours, then wake up and can't get back to sleep. Among the causes to look for are obstructive sleep apnea and nocturnal myoclonus, both mentioned previously. Another possibility is a sudden drop in blood sugar, most often caused by eating sweets or drinking alcohol in the evening. The blood sugar drop and resulting release of adrenaline to bring the blood sugar level back up are often interpreted as a nightmare or night terror. It may help to remind yourself that there is really nothing to be afraid of, even to explain the low-blood-sugar-adrenaline-rush phenomenon to yourself again as you work to calm yourself down.

Sleep specialists consider one or two wakings per night, and even one or two trips to the bathroom, as within the normal range. Often people wake up, look at the clock, and start worrying that they cannot get back to sleep, which makes matters worse. I've learned to look at the clock (I can't resist, although I wish I could), and if it's one or two in the morning, I tell myself, "I have four or five hours before I have to get up. I have all that time to lie here, enjoy my thoughts, and be responsible for nothing." If necessary, I repeat all the muscle-loosening techniques I did before I fell asleep, and do the mental self-talk and picture-making activities I mentioned above. These days I usually get back to sleep.

It's somewhat harder, but still possible, to be unperturbed when I wake up at three or four in the morning. Blood sugar levels are at their lowest then, causing us to feel more pessimistic and depressed than at other times. It's quite a challenge to control my thoughts. Sometimes I remind myself how lucky I am not to have to light the fire in the stove and go milk the cows, as some of my neighbors still do. If I can get comfortable just lying in bed and resting, that's what I do. If I'm still awake after an hour or so and no longer enjoy relaxing in the quiet night, I usually get out of bed and start my day. However, I sometimes get my deepest sleep between five and six, when the radio goes on and my day officially begins.

• • • • Moving in Bed and • • • • Getting Out of Bed

Some people find when they learn to sleep soundly that moving in their sleep wakes them with pain and stiffness. Others say they still wake up stiff and sore in the morning, but that these sensations disappear when they have moved around a bit. These things happen because it is in the nature of fibromyalgic muscles to stiffen and "gel" when we're not moving. To minimize discomfort, try these suggestions:

• Anytime you come to sufficient consciousness during the night, stretch before you shift to a new position, and make it your business to find a new position before going back to sleep. You will find this avoids much pain and stiffness.

• When you move in bed, roll with your head down; don't lead with your head, which places great strain on your neck. Use your arms and legs to help you move.

• Yawn and stretch in the morning before you get out of bed. When you yawn, if you can pause a bit after the in-breath before letting it out, you'll provide more oxygen to your blood and brain, helping you to feel alert and fresh sooner.

• To get out of bed, roll onto your side, facing the edge of the bed. Pull your knees up toward your chest, then drop your feet over the side of the bed, pushing on the bed with your topside hand and using the weight of your feet and lower body to get you to a sitting position. Pause for a moment once you're sitting. Then lean forward and let your head down between your knees. Don't push; just let the weight of your head do the work. This way, you'll stretch out your spine and back muscles and make standing up much easier.

• • • • • • • • • • • • • • • • • • •

6

Committed Relationships

Fibromyalgia is tough on couples. I know of no statistics on the subject, but the hundreds of conversations I've had with people who have fibromyalgia give me the impression that more divorces occur among couples in which one member has FM than in the general population. In this chapter we'll look at things that can go wrong between couples, and what we can do to head off problems or make repairs. Although I'll be focusing on conventional marriages, the ideas apply just as well to other long-term relationships.

Everything changes when one member of a committed partnership becomes chronically ill—roles, the division of labor, and plans for the future are altered no matter how we try to maintain our normal patterns of thought and behavior. The more the partners are committed to the traditional male-female roles, the more difficult it is to accept and adapt to these changes. Learning to adjust to the new circumstances demands both strength and flexibility.

Emotional Strains

Try as we might to be rational about our life roles, we all have expectations of ourselves and our partners. Exceptions exist, of course, but most women see themselves as the primary care-givers in the family, most men as the primary breadwinners, even if the women work and the men change diapers. Fibro-myalgia plays havoc with these roles and expectations. A man who has FM may find himself forced to stay home and assume unfamiliar responsibilities while his wife goes out to work. The woman who is ill needs care herself. She needs relief from her usual household tasks, at least until she can develop new tech-niques to handle those that aren't completely impossible. She may become unable to hold an outside job, something both she and her husband had expected of her. The economic conse-quences may be serious, possibly requiring her husband to take on a second job.

Shirley and Jim are one such couple. Because she is unable to work, Shirley's financial contribution comes from Social Se-curity disability payments, which dropped to $64 a month when she and Jim married. Jim has two jobs and works seventy to seventy-five hours a week to make ends meet. "I've seen Jim work twenty-five days in a row, putting in more than ten hours a day," Shirley says. "This is very frustrating," Jim adds. "I have a quick temper when I get stressed, which seems to happen almost every other day. I think it's almost as bad for Shirley, because she sees me putting forth so much effort to keep us housed, fed, and clothed." The problem is no less severe, of course, if the person with FM is the husband.

All kinds of emotions come into play: resentment, anger, frustration, guilt, anxiety, fear, sadness, grief, depression—and, perhaps the worst of all, isolation. It's easy to understand why the person with fibromyalgia would have these feelings, but it's important to remember that the healthy party is subject to the same emotions. Each partner needs to air his or her feelings in a supportive and validating atmosphere. In some relation-ships the partners can provide this atmosphere for each other. In others, the feelings are too painful to be said or heard, and professional counseling is needed.

Living with a chronically ill person is enormously difficult. Some people find the role of caregiver to be demeaning and without status. During a fibromyalgia flare, the healthy mate may be called on to do the work of both partners, working a full day and then coming home to make dinner, clean up, and do a load of laundry. This kind of burden can easily provoke resentment. The one who needs care may feel guilty about being unable to live up to his or her normal responsibilities. It's easy to imagine the person with FM resenting the need to ask for help, and looking for signs that the spouse is running out of patience. Carla, a forty-year-old former practical nurse, feels that her inability to do housework is putting a strain on her marriage. She says her husband "resents having to do all the cleaning and cooking and shopping. He doesn't verbalize this, but I feel it."

Both partners may experience fear. The ill spouse fears that the healthy partner will grow weary of the situation and leave. Meanwhile, the healthy one is afraid that things will get even worse, or that all the responsibilities will prove to be too much. The couple's social life suffers, leaving them isolated from their friends. Unfortunately, each partner may be so wrapped up in his or her own feelings and thoughts that the other person's needs fade into the background. That leads to the worst kind of isolation of all, the inability to express all these feelings and find comfort.

Singly and together, the couple needs time to grieve for what has been lost. Sean, the healthy husband of a woman with FM, says, "Laura was very active when I first met her. Now she's a shell of who she was. I watch her struggle constantly with a constellation of symptoms and problems that no healthy person will ever experience. Do you have any idea how hard this is on the spouse?"

Sean explains his pain and frustration in terms that anyone who ever had a pet can understand: "What if you had to watch the beloved family collie, more human than dog, hobbling around in pain from a displaced hip, knowing there was nothing you could do to help with the pain? It's an awful feeling to watch the one you love suffer almost constantly."

Both Sean and Laura have experienced losses, which must

be mourned. It's not easy for him to say, or for her to hear, that he misses his evenings out with his buddies. It's hard for her to admit, and for him to accept, that she grieves for her hard-won independence and her place in the working world. If left unacknowledged, such losses will fester and cause ever-increasing pain. Each individual wants to hear the other person say, "I know. I'm sorry."

Defensiveness and attempts to belittle the other's pain are inappropriate and self-defeating. If you think you hear blame in your partner's voice, try to test your perception. Say something like this: "I get the feeling that you think there's something I could have done to avoid this situation. I'm probably being oversensitive, but I thought I'd better check with you."

Even when the healthy partner starts out being supportive, the long-term nature of fibromyalgia can have a corrosive effect on the couple's relationship. Joe was patient and supportive when Helen got her diagnosis, joining her in the search for information on the Internet and encouraging her to come to terms with the understanding that she would always have fibromyalgia. But after a while, Joe ran out of patience. "You know what it is now," he told Helen. "It's time you just learned to live with it." Stung by Joe's insensitive remark, Helen visited a counselor, who assured her that it was perfectly normal to feel depressed and grieve over the loss of good health. With the counselor's encouragement, Helen joined a local FM support group, where she found help in coming to terms with her diagnosis and an outlet for all the things she wanted to say about fibromyalgia. "I decided it was in the best interest of my marriage not to dwell constantly on the subject in talking with Joe," she says.

Before she dropped the subject, though, Helen and Joe had a serious talk in which Helen admitted she felt "defective" and was frightened of her future. She asked Joe if he wanted to leave her. "He seemed appalled by the idea and told me he had married me for better or worse, in sickness and in health, and had no intention of leaving me," she says. Still, Helen sought Joe's reassurance several times more before she could believe Joe meant what he said. "It's taken time to adjust, but once I became better able to push thoughts of FM more to the side and not have it dominate my life, things have become easier. Joe has told me he feels I've become 'me' again, albeit with some new limitations."

Sexual Intimacy

The grief that comes from a decrease in sexual activity may be the hardest pain of all to acknowledge and discuss. When pain comes on the scene, sexual desire often disappears. Mood-altering drugs, even at the low doses commonly prescribed for people with fibromyalgia, can blunt sexual interest and ability. Having been diagnosed with a chronic illness is a blow to your self-image that may leave you feeling unattractive sexually. Add to that the distraction that pain causes and the fear that sexual activity will cause damage or injury, and you have the recipe for serious trouble.

Many of us have attitudes about sex that work against a satisfactory resolution of sexual dysfunction. We equate sex with intercourse. We demand that sex be spontaneous and think it won't be nearly as much fun if we plan for it. We believe sexual activity must always culminate in orgasm. By taking these narrow views of our own sexuality and that of our partner, we deprive ourselves of a great deal of pleasure. How much better off we are if we examine our thoughts and beliefs about sexuality and change those that are getting in the way of our satisfaction. (See below on healthy beliefs about sexuality.)

• Healthy Beliefs About Sexuality •

• Sex is not a contest. Pleasure, not performance, is the point of it.

- Intercourse is a part of sex, not the whole thing.

- Stroking, kissing, and cuddling are important in themselves, not just a means to an end.

- Lack of an erection or orgasm does not signal the absence of love.

- There can be plenty of fun without orgasms.

- It's OK to ask for what you want, and to say what gives you discomfort or pain.

• •

Most people find it hard to ask for sexual attention, fearing they will be rebuffed. Yet waiting to be asked, while good for self-protection, can be disastrous when one of the partners has fibromyalgia. For most fibromyalgics, one side effect of medication, pain, and fatigue is the loss of that delicious sexy feeling that happens at odd moments and makes it possible to risk initiating an encounter. This poses a dilemma for the healthy partner: Does that partner make his or her wants known without regard to how the other party is feeling, or suffer in silence?

Edna and Tom struggled with such issues for fifteen years before they separated. Edna says illness was "lurking in the background" when she and Tom married. He accepted her four children from a previous marriage as his own. But soon after their wedding, pain and weakness took center stage. "We were very much in love and very close," Edna recalls, "but as the years went by and I kept getting sicker, Tom started pulling away from me. I began to suspect that he was repelled by my illness." After seven years, during which doctors "passed it off as stress," Edna was diagnosed with fibromyalgia. Edna says Tom told her "if I would just get my attitude adjusted, I would get better. I needed comfort and support from him, but I didn't let him know clearly enough, nor was he able to tell what I needed. I felt ashamed of being sick, like I had failed in some way."

By this time, Edna had lost all interest in sex. "He has high needs, and I have low-to-no needs," she says. "I was always feeling pressure, and he was always feeling guilty for making demands." Tom, whose work as an engineer required a great deal of travel, became emotionally involved with another woman. "Something inside of me died then, and I began to resent him," Edna says. She delivered an ultimatum: "He had to make the decision either to work on healing our marriage or leave. He chose to leave." After more than a year's separation, during which Edna filed for divorce, Tom approached her about a reconciliation. "I am satisfied with the growth he has made. He admits to being unsupportive and not contributing to the family emotionally. I want to heal my family," says Edna.

Edna isn't sure a reconciliation will work. Tom's emphasis on the importance of her orgasm—"something I don't need and don't really want," she says—remains a source of friction. "I'm concerned about the extreme fragility of my body and the pain rolling around in bed will cause. I wish we could just be together, be companions on the journey of life. I just wish I could get some affection without it leading to having to per-form."

Asked if she can imagine Tom's point of view, Edna says, "I think it must make him feel sad and unwanted. If those needs are there, he can't help it any more than I can help not having them. That matters to me." Edna grants both sets of needs equal importance, but resents the fact that she is seen as the one with the problem. "We both want to reconcile and have both committed to being honest with each other about every-thing."

Some couples find inventive ways to work out such prob-lems. In the early years of their marriage, before Martha's FM diagnosis, when Eric suggested, by word or deed, that they make love, Martha would often respond favorably and then change her mind, saying she didn't feel well enough. To Eric, the disappointment was "worse than a flat-out refusal." Later, when she understood why her pain and energy levels varied so widely, Martha learned not to make promises she couldn't keep. Instead, the couple made a standing date to meet in bed every Sunday afternoon, when Martha's pain and fatigue are usually at their lowest. Nothing is allowed to interfere with their time together. There is no commitment beyond that. Nobody has to promise to do anything. They just lock the doors, shut off the telephone, get into their nightclothes, and snuggle, focusing their attention on the physical sensation of closeness. Usually, Martha expects nothing more to happen, and both are pleasantly surprised when she responds to Eric's stroking. Sometimes they don't get past the caressing stage, but the warmth of each other's bodies and the tacit expression of love and respect fuel them for the week.

Contrary to cultural myth, making a date to make love can actually add to the fun. Normally shy and reserved, Martha finds herself flirting with Eric the day before their date. Eric loves the attention and flirts back. "If you don't consider intercourse as the only valid form of sex, there's more sex in our lives now than ever before," Eric says.

Dialogue

To be successful in their marriage, couples need to be good communicators. This need increases dramatically when chronic illness adds stress to the relationship. Some people are open and honest to a fault. They have no problem speaking up when their partner displeases or disappoints them, believing that instant feedback is the only way to rectify the situation. Others hold back on expressing annoyance or dissatisfaction, hoping to keep the peace. Eventually such people risk building a wall of resentment around themselves, with toxic effects on the relationship. Neither constant confrontation nor constant denial is in the best interests of people who value the relationship they are in.

Good timing is an art that anyone can learn. If someone is stepping on your toe or pressing on a tender point, it's appropriate to speak up right away. But if the hurt is of a more abstract nature, sometimes it's a good idea to acknowledge the feeling to yourself, waiting for a better time to mention it and seek corrective action. Look at it this way: He said something that hurt you. What do you want to do about it? Do you want to hurt him back, or to let him know how and why it hurt so he won't do it again? Surely, since you value your relationship, revenge is not your motive; corrective action is. The best time to make a correction is when the other person is able to hear what you have to say. A spouse returning home tired after a day's work is in no condition to hear criticism and react in a calm and rational manner. A person in the midst of a fibromyalgia flare-up has enough to deal with without facing confrontation. The key to successful communication is to find a time when you can speak in a rational, nonblaming way and your partner can listen without feeling defensive. Some couples find that the mellow time after a sexual engagement works well, but the timing is a highly personal matter and one you may want to discuss with your partner—preferably when you're both feeling good about life in general.

Most people have difficulty giving and receiving negative feedback. You may have been taught to think it wrong to express your needs, feelings, and opinions. You may have the idea that a negative message is a sign of disapproval and dislike. If this is so, you would do well to reconsider. The basis of a mutually successful relationship is mutual honesty, delivered in a peaceful and constructive manner. It does a relationship no good at all for one or both members to keep hidden their wants and needs and to store up hurts rather than seek a way to heal them. In a sense, behavior that avoids conflict at all costs is dishonest. It gives the other person the impression that all is well when it isn't. Some amount of conflict is the inevitable result of two people living together. Eternal peace and harmony is not the way the world works.

The secret of a successful relationship is the establishment of an informal set of procedures that allow the parties to express themselves without being punitive or threatening, and to hear each other's expressions without feeling punished or threatened. This is the difference between assertive behavior and aggression. Assertive behavior is a set of skills that include the ability to make requests, say no, express opinions, disclose wants and needs, and show both affection and displeasure. An assertive person is easier, not harder, to live with than one whose feelings are kept hidden. With an assertive person, you need never fear an explosion of negative emotion long bottled up. Situations are dealt with in a timely and appropriate manner. The response is in proportion to the stimulus. An assertive person is a full partner in the relationship. With someone who keeps feelings hidden, there is an unequal balance of power. He or she may be the more submissive partner, but it is just as likely that the other person will sense the underlying negativity and live in fear of an explosion. No one should have to be afraid of the person he or she lives with. Assertiveness is a skill that anyone can learn and that everyone should learn.

Assertiveness is the constructive expression of negative feelings such as anger or dissatisfaction. This expression is accomplished calmly, without anger or blame. It consists of describing a situation, explaining what is wrong with the situation, and, if possible, suggesting a course of action to remedy it. A successful assertion avoids imputing motives and avoids evoking a defensive response in the listener. The typical assertion has three components:

1. A statement of the undesired behavior, beginning with "When you . . ."
2. A statement of feeling, beginning with "I feel . . ."
3. A statement of the negative consequences, such as, "Because . . ."

It may also include a statement of the desired change, in a sentence beginning "I would like . . ."

Meeting Each Other's Needs

Here is an example of a source of friction between Rona, who has FM, and Thad, who does not. Like many people with FM, Rona tends to be poorly coordinated, tripping over objects that others successfully avoid, even when she sees them. Thad is an almost ideal partner for Rona, except for one fact: He has a high tolerance for clutter and tends to leave things where they fall. When her back isn't acting up, Rona will bend over, pick up Thad's belongings, and put them away, grumbling to herself all the time. But sometimes she can't bend over, doesn't notice an item that Thad has dropped on the floor, and ends up tripping on it. This pattern has been going on for years.

One day, while Thad is at work, Rona trips over a shoe he left on the stairs. She could have hurt herself badly if she hadn't been holding on to the railing. Furious, Rona works off her anger in a cleaning spree, during which she picks up everything Thad has left lying around and piles it on his side of the bed. His dirty socks she puts on his pillow to ensure that he won't miss the point. By the time Thad comes home, Rona is physically exhausted, emotionally spent, and stretched out on the living room sofa, a damp cloth on her forehead. "Hi, honey," he calls from the front door, then stops short as he sees Rona. She hasn't looked this bad in months. "What happened?" he asks, genuine concern in his voice.

"I nearly killed myself tripping over your damn shoe," Rona replies, her voice somewhere between a snarl and a whine. "I pulled a muscle in my shoulder but didn't realize it until I finished cleaning up your mess. It's obvious you don't care at all about my safety. I'm tired of being your maid, and I want you to clean up after yourself from now on—or else!"

Thad wisely declines to explore what the "else" might be, but that's the limit to his wisdom. He replies, "Look, Rona. I work hard all day, and you're home doing nothing. If I happen to leave something lying around, you can bloody well make yourself useful by picking it up. That's not too much to ask."

What we have here is a recipe for warfare. Rona must now remind Thad that she'd love to be going out and being among people the way he is, but she tires too easily and has too much pain. Thad can reply that if she pulled herself together and got some exercise she wouldn't hurt so much. He can raise the ante by pointing out how much weight she's gained lying around doing nothing and suggest that if she weren't so fat she wouldn't be so clumsy. She can cry; he can storm out to the corner pub for a beer with his buddies. They can both do without dinner or grab leftovers and heat them in the microwave oven. He can leave his dishes in the sink and his underwear on top of the clothes hamper. She can throw them in the trash. He can be snoring enthusiastically by the time she comes to bed. She can stare at the ceiling all night long, enraged at his lack of feelings for her. The possibilities are endless.

Of course, it need not be this way. Thad grew up in a home where his mother picked up after everybody without complaint. During his bachelor years he left things lying around all over his apartment. Until now, it never entered his mind that Rona had a problem with his habits. Had he been paying attention, he might have noticed some mild displeasure on Rona's part, but she never said a word.

Let's roll the tape back and start again. We'll have to select a time earlier in their relationship, long before Thad grew to expect Rona to pick up after him without feeling imposed upon, and long before Rona developed the rage that erupted into an exhausting cleanup campaign. We'll have Rona pick up one of Thad's shoes off the step and put it on her side of the bed to remind her to speak with him about it when the time is right. That evening, while they're getting ready for bed, she says, "Honey, when you leave your things lying around the house, I feel annoyed because, for one thing, I sometimes trip over things even though I see them in my path. Besides, it makes me feel that you don't value my time and energy, and I'm sensitive about that since I can't go out and earn money and contribute the way you do. I'd like to find a way for both of us to feel comfortable about this. What do you think about a box for you to throw things into when you don't feel like putting them away?"

Thad's reaction will almost certainly be quite different. He won't have to defend himself, because Rona isn't blaming him for anything. She's simply stating as clearly as possible how she sees the situation and how she feels about it. She expresses annoyance, not anger, because she hasn't been piling irritation upon irritation until it spilled over into fury. She's told him how she feels, and why. She has indicated a wish to resolve the problem so that both partners are satisfied. And she's even offered a suggested solution in a way that gives Thad the opportunity to modify or replace it. The suggestion is optional, but the expression of a wish to make things better is not. What the suggestion does, though, is give Thad a way to respond without needing to defend himself or come up with his own solution. Since Rona has obviously given this matter some thought and Thad probably has not, it's appropriate for her to make the first suggestion, as long as she leaves Thad a way to improve upon it.

Does this example ring a bell with you? Is there a hidden bone of contention in your domestic life that you'd like to dig up and, with your partner, chew over? If so, think the issue through and plan your strategy. Be prepared to:

- Bring up the subject at a time when neither of you is over-tired or stressed, and when there is sufficient time to do justice to the discussion.
- State the issue in neutral terms.
- Describe how you feel about it.
- Say why you feel that way.

- Say what you'd like to see happen.
- Offer a solution, if you can.

When the time comes and you start the discussion, you may be surprised at how well this technique works. If it is the polar opposite of your normal way of expressing displeasure, however, be prepared for your partner to be a bit unsettled at first. You may have to take this approach a few times on a few different issues before he or she trusts you not to shift gears in mid-conversation and turn it into an argument. Be trustworthy, and you will become trusted.

Of course, the technique isn't going to work if one member of the partnership denies or is unaware of the fact that the other has needs. It's easy to forget about another person's needs when you're all wrapped up in pain. It's just as easy to forget when you're so burdened with financial worries, work pressures, and the added responsibility for work around the house that comes with being the healthy spouse of a person with fibromyalgia. An added problem in any marriage is that most of us have been taught to place a high value on independence. We tend to confuse being independent with being without needs. Often the only acceptable need is the need for sex. But none of us is really without needs. We need to feel loved, appreciated, and cared for. We need to share our feelings and experiences with someone who will validate them. We need to be recognized for our achievements and receive sympathy for our defeats. We need to feel physically and emotionally safe in our own homes, and more.

Many times, a marital quarrel results when both individuals are competing to get their needs met, and neither is meeting the other's needs. We feel let down and angry, although we are probably unaware of the real cause of our anger and therefore blame it on the other person. Joan, a consultant whose job involves travel, tells of the times when she would come home from a business trip "feeling exhausted and bruised because of my need to appear normal when I don't feel that way."

Thomas, a programmer who works at home, had been alone for several days with nothing but the dog and cat for company. "Tommy would pick me up at the airport, and within moments we'd be fighting over something that is utterly stupid. The reason? I'd want to be told how happy he is to have me home. He'd want to hear all about the trip because he wants to share that part of my life. And that's the last thing I want to talk about. But none of this would get said. What we'd say is a lot of stupid, childish stuff."

Eventually, Joan realized that "what was going on was a whole bunch of needs banging up against a whole other bunch of needs." She suggested that she and Thomas do "a quick neediness check as soon as we get into the car. We find we can quite readily agree on who is the needier, and that person gets 'taken care of' first. We both love each other enough to be able to put our own needs on hold when we see that the other is even needier. It works out fine, and we haven't fought when I came home from a trip for several years now."

Joan and Thomas have worked out the kind of relationship that Ernesto Vasquez, M.D., a psychiatrist in Columbus, Ohio, referred to at a fibromyalgia conference in 1997. A healthy relationship, he said, is one in which "both partners consistently try to meet each other's needs in a reciprocal manner." That's a goal worth striving for. With patience and goodwill, it can be achieved.

7

Mind and Body

Fibromyalgia is a multifaceted illness. It has a profound effect on us both physically and mentally. But at the same time, our physical and mental states have a profound effect on our fibromyalgia. In other words, FM puts us in a bad place physically and mentally, but being in a bad place physically and mentally makes our FM worse. This chapter will help you reverse the downward spiral of pain and depression.

If you are like most people who have fibromyalgia, you have been told by at least one doctor that the problem is all in your mind. It's no wonder we resist the idea that our minds have anything at all to do with the problem. However, that is exactly the proposition of this chapter: What goes on in your mind did *not* cause your symptoms, but it is the single most important factor in improving the quality of your life. Furthermore, I hope to convince you that you have a great deal of power over what you think and how you feel, and that you can use that power to make your life richer and more rewarding.

When I was a teen, the cultural craze was a book called *The Power of Positive Thinking*, by Norman Vincent Peale. Following the author's advice, my grandfather used to come to the breakfast table every morning and announce, "Day by day, in every way, I'm getting better and better." When I asked why he said that, he explained that people's thoughts can influence how they feel, and that since he was healthy and wanted to stay that way he was using his mind to help him maintain good health.

Dr. Peale was years ahead of science in this insight, but today it has been amply demonstrated that the connections in our brains that carry our thoughts become strengthened by repeated use. Just as you can learn to twirl a baton or play the piano by practicing the same motions over and over again, so, too, do you develop habits of thought by thinking along the same lines repeatedly. You can choose to allow yourself to reinforce either positive or negative thoughts.

Perhaps the idea that you can choose what you think is new to you, but it's true. You can also choose, to a very great extent, how to feel about what you think. Today there is a large body of research data and clinical experience to show that people can learn to control their moods by applying a few relatively simple mental techniques and principles. If you haven't yet experienced the power of controlling your own thoughts and feelings, I envy you; you are on the brink of a breakthrough discovery. I won't ask you to believe me until you have proven it to yourself. I simply ask that you suspend disbelief, that you take a neutral attitude toward this proposition and give it a chance to prove itself to you.

Mental Responses to Pain

To say that pain is unpleasant is putting it mildly. No mental power or change of attitude is ever going to make pain anything but unpleasant. But pain has another attribute over which we can exercise control. Pain is frightening. We are taught from infancy that we should be afraid of pain. If we were colicky babies, our cries of pain probably made our parents frantic, and they could not have avoided communicating to us their grief and frustration at being unable to provide relief. To a dependent child, a parent's negative feelings are frightening, so our association between pain and fright may go back to our earliest days. Later, when we were learning to walk and fell down, an adult would scoop us up when we cried and make a fuss as a way to comfort us—a normal, loving reaction to the pain of our falling. Some of us had parents who said things such as "Don't run so fast. You'll fall and hurt yourself," so we learned to fear pain as the result of motion. When we were ill with an earache, perhaps, or a bellyache, we learned that pain means something is definitely wrong, that our lives would be disrupted for a period of time, and that the adults around us would be upset.

This is not said to blame the people who cared for us as we were growing up. It is the responsibility of adults to protect children, and that involves a considerable amount of warning and fretting to make a child safe and protected, and to teach reasonable, life-saving caution. It would be a pitiful child, indeed, who was surrounded by people indifferent to his or her pain. But in the process of performing as responsible adults, those around us contributed to the perception that pain is invariably a sign of danger or misery. Thus, pain becomes for most of us more than unpleasant. It becomes something to fear.

Pain causes stress on two levels. It is stressful in itself, but it is also stressful because of the fear it induces. Pain has yet another harmful characteristic. It causes stiffness and tension in the part of the body where it occurs. It is a normal human reaction to tighten our muscles when we feel pain. Think of what you do when you feel a shooting pain or muscle cramp. I'll bet you tense up instinctively and hold the painful part rigid, trying not to move it for fear of causing more pain. This reaction makes perfectly good sense, given what we have learned about pain in the course of our lives—that pain's message is we must react to protect ourselves.

But one of the proven facts about fibromyalgia is that we have more than an NDA (person Not Diagnosed with Anything) does of substance P, the chemical that tells our brains we have pain. Most people with fibromyalgia have had the experience of crying out from pain only to be told by someone observing the scene that such a little stimulus couldn't possibly have caused that much pain. But you know it did; you're not a sissy. In fact, you're probably better than most people at concealing your pain, because you've had so much of it.

Next time pain captures your attention, try this: Focus on the place that hurts. Notice how tense and tight it is. Try to tune in to what you're thinking about the pain. Tell yourself that this particular pain is just pain for its own sake; it doesn't mean something is torn or broken or infected or inflamed. Tell yourself it's a muscle spasm (unless you know otherwise, it probably is) and that you can fix it. Close your eyes if you can, and concentrate on loosening the painful area. You may need to first tighten it even more, to get in touch with the muscles you want to control. Try to liberate the pain from its central location and let it spread out throughout your body. Picture the most painful spot as a circle of red and watch that circle lose its clearly defined shape and become a blur. Remember that there was only so much red to begin with, and as it spreads notice how the red fades to pink as it covers a larger area with the same amount of pigment. Keep your muscles as loose as possible; don't let fear and anxiety tighten you up.

As you become proficient in this technique, you will find that the pain becomes less sharp and demanding of your attention. Once you have that level of control, you can move on to the next step, which is to deprive the pain of your attention by engaging in some other activity. If you can, exercise the area. That's the best activity. Strong muscles hurt less than weak muscles.

The important point here is that fear and anxiety accentuate pain. If you can get your emotions under control, you will have taken a giant step toward controlling your pain. Let's look at other ways we can control our thoughts and feelings to improve the quality of our lives.

Mood and Stress

···

The ideal mental training for people with fibromyalgia is a technique known as cognitive behavioral therapy (CBT), sometimes called cognitive therapy. Developed at the University of Pennsylvania's School of Medicine in the 1970s by a psychiatrist, Aaron T. Beck, M.D., CBT has been used experimentally with people who have fibromyalgia, with beneficial results.[10] CBT experiments have also involved patients with chronic fatigue syndrome and rheumatoid arthritis. Generally, the findings are that people who use CBT achieve significantly greater relief from pain than those who do relaxation exercises. Speaking to a patient conference in 1997, Daniel Clauw, M.D., a leading FM researcher, called cognitive behavioral therapy "the single most effective treatment" for FM. CBT helps patients develop a sense of control over the situation, he explained, adding, "Improvement comes when people develop a sense of control, when they come to understand what they can do to make it better and what makes it worse."

People who are severely depressed may do best if they have some sessions with a cognitive behavioral therapist. Contact the Center for Cognitive Therapy, listed in the "Resources" section of this book, for the names of therapists trained in this technique.

Many people with FM can do the work of cognitive therapy by themselves, with guidance from a book. *Feeling Good,* by David D. Burns, M.D., who studied with Dr. Beck, is designed specifically for this purpose. The rest of this section draws heavily on that book and is intended to help you start thinking along CBT lines. If what you read in this section makes sense to you, I urge you to learn more about CBT.

Cognitive behavioral therapy is based on the premise that people who are depressed or anxious are thinking in a negative manner that causes them to act in a self-defeating way. CBT holds that people can train themselves to eliminate these negative thought patterns, stop acting against their own best interests, and gain more self-confidence and self-respect. The training doesn't take very long, and it has been shown in many cases to be more effective than medicine in relieving depression. This doesn't mean that you should stop taking an antidepressant if one is currently prescribed for you, but it does mean that you may be able to avoid taking one if you haven't started and that your need for antidepressants may be reduced if you are taking them.

Please understand that I'm not saying CBT will cure your fibromyalgia, or that depression, anxiety, or self-defeating thoughts are the cause of your FM. Many people with fibromyalgia are depressed, but depression is no more prevalent in FM than in other patient populations, such as those with multiple sclerosis or rheumatoid arthritis. Until you know enough about your condition to experience some control over it, anxiety about your future is a natural response. Self-defeating thoughts are the result of anxiety and depression, and these thoughts perpetuate the condition, but they didn't cause it. However, when you can rid yourself of these demons, you will feel much better and your life will be headed in the direction you choose, rather than the one your negative emotions dictate.

The first principle of cognitive therapy is that your mood is determined by your thoughts, perceptions, attitudes, and beliefs. You feel the way you do right this minute because of the thoughts you are thinking. For example, if you are thinking that this can't be right, that it's just another trick to get your hopes up and then disappoint you, you are feeling down and discouraged. But if this idea makes some sense to you and you're thinking it's worth exploring because it may prove helpful, you're feeling somewhat more hopeful and upbeat. Whichever set of thoughts you're having, where do you think they come from? From you, of course. Nobody controls your mind but you. You choose which thoughts to have and, to a great extent, you can choose how you will feel.

The second principle is that when you are feeling depressed

or anxious, your thoughts are dominated by negativity. Everything is gloomy, there is no hope, and you tend to feel that things have always been this way. If you look into your past, you see only the bad things that have happened, and you can't imagine a future that holds anything but problems and pain. You are convinced that you will always feel as hopeless or anxiety-ridden as you do now.

The third principle is that these negative thoughts almost always are based on distortions of fact. Cognitive behavioral therapy teaches us to recognize these distortions and eliminate them from our thinking. As you do this, you begin to think more rationally and objectively. You gain control over your thoughts and feel better. Although CBT won't cure your fibromyalgia, it can enhance your ability to manage and cope with it. Remember that stress and depression exaggerate pain.

Depression and anxiety aren't the only emotions that CBT can help you to relieve. Anger is another. CBT can teach you how to find alternative interpretations for the events and kinds of behavior that make you angry. That can have a profound effect on your fibromyalgia. Anger is a particularly harmful stressor for people who have fibromyalgia. There is growing evidence that people with FM have inadequate adrenal systems. Allowing ourselves to get angry calls forth adrenaline surges that we can ill afford. Most of us feel ill, foggy, and depressed in the wake of an adrenaline-producing episode. It's an experience we want to avoid. Anger, like all emotions, comes not from the event itself so much as from the way we interpret the event. It may not be possible to avoid all negative emotions, but the power that comes with the ability to control our reactions is enormously effective in improving our health and the quality of our lives.

One of the things CBT teaches is that we all have certain automatic thoughts that pop into our minds in response to certain stimuli. For example, suppose you forget to pay a bill on time and the company adds a penalty fee onto the next month's bill. One automatic thought might be, "I never do anything right." If you can stop yourself from generalizing this way, you will recognize that this one thing you didn't do right doesn't wipe out all the many things you've done right in your life. Or suppose you're stuck in traffic on the way to a meeting. What might the automatic thoughts be? Perhaps you think, "I'm always late." Or "Everybody at the meeting will think I'm irresponsible." But if you reflect, you can surely think of many times you've been punctual. You can hardly expect yourself to predict when a traffic jam will occur. And assuming you've arrived on time for the last three meetings, the people at this one will hardly give your tardiness a thought unless you come in looking like a whipped dog and call attention to yourself by talking in great detail about the traffic. Identifying your own automatic thoughts and replacing them with more realistic ideas is something you can learn to do, starting right now.

Perhaps you are wondering, if negative emotions play such an important role in fibromyalgia, what is the relationship between feelings and the brain chemicals we have been told are out of balance in people who have fibromyalgia? Here is one explanation: Anxiety, depression, and anger all cause stress. Stress depletes the brain chemical serotonin. Depleted serotonin is associated with elevated substance P. Elevated substance P increases the perception of pain. Pain causes anxiety, depression, and anger. Also, depleted serotonin interferes with sleep. Dysfunctional sleep causes pain. Pain causes anxiety, depression, and anger. So you see how a negative cycle is established when the brain plays host to negative emotions.

You could just as well describe the cycle by beginning with serotonin. Measurement of serotonin in the brain, where it is active, involves invasive procedures that physicians and scientists are reluctant to perform for research purposes, so instead they measure the presence of serotonin's metabolic by-product, called 5-HIAA, in the spinal fluid. Since they find less of serotonin's breakdown product, it is reasonable to assume that people with fibromyalgia have less serotonin to begin with.[11]

It's pointless to try to figure out whether lack of serotonin causes the physical and emotional symptoms of FM or whether the symptoms of FM cause a lack of serotonin. The two almost certainly feed on each other. What makes sense for those who want to improve the way they feel, physically and mentally, is to break into the cycle at the easiest and most convenient place. For most of us, that place is the intellectual and emotional plane. Whether or not you take mood-altering drugs, learning to control your own mental reactions to events in your life will contribute enormously to your health and well-being.

One of the techniques I use to relieve anxiety is to ask myself the question "What's the worst that can happen?" Anxiety is a shapeless mass of feelings that include fear, dread, and worry. I find that if I define what I fear, dread, or worry about, I can invariably control those emotions and make the anxiety go away. For example, it is a matter of pride for me, as a writer of magazine articles, that I have never missed a deadline. Still, after more than twenty years working as a writer, at some point in almost every assignment I find myself gripped with anxiety that this will be the first time I miss my deadline. Intellectually, I know that editors always set deadlines with plenty of slack, so that if the writer submits inferior work or misses a given date they have time to fix the article or fill in with another one. Emotionally, however, my deadline sometimes looms in front of me like a monster so huge that I can't see its edges. That's when I ask myself the question. It always turns out that the worst that can happen isn't nearly so bad, once I give it a shape and look straight at it. (Anxiety or panic attacks are a separate problem that can often be solved by an adjustment in diet and nutrition, a subject that comes up in the next chapter.)

Many people with fibromyalgia seek adrenaline-producing situations to combat fatigue. The hormone is a potent brain chemical. It is associated with the "fight or flight" response that one experiences in an emergency. Secreted by the adrenal glands, one of which is found on each kidney, adrenaline (epinephrine is another name for it) makes the heart beat faster, speeding blood to the brain and other organs. It raises the blood sugar level, providing added energy for a fast response. Obviously, the ability to produce adrenaline in response to danger can be a lifesaving mechanism. Unfortunately, the feeling can be addictive for people. If you find this hard to believe, hang out for a while in a video game arcade and observe the behavior of the players.

Running on adrenaline is extremely counterproductive. No one can run on adrenaline forever, and those of us with fibromyalgia tend to be deficient in the chemical, so that when we stop pumping adrenaline we experience exhaustion, malaise, and often mental confusion. Learning to control adrenaline surges was an important step for me in gaining control over my FM.

I mentioned this phenomenon once in a fibromyalgia discussion group on the Internet. (See the "Resources" section for Internet addresses and information.) The response was amazing. People wrote saying that they couldn't get along without pumping adrenaline. One man wrote, "The only time I feel alive is when I'm high on adrenaline." Only a few recognized the aftereffects of an adrenaline surge and tried to avoid such stimulating situations.

If you recognize in yourself a tendency to anger over things that others consider unimportant, consider the possibility that adrenaline is at work. I've seen "flame wars" on the Internet—verbal arguments over trivia—where people with FM were involved, and I could imagine the participants sitting at their computers, furious with the messages addressed to them, and fighting back with vigor. If they paused to think about it, they would probably realize how unimportant these arguments are, and find another, less harmful way to feel energetic.

Ask yourself if you fit this profile. Do you find yourself getting "charged up" in response to things in your environment or just to keep your energy up? Don't you find that you feel worse after an adrenaline surge? If you determine that adrena-

line is a factor in your illness, there are some things you can do
to gain control over this physical response to stress:

• See if you can detect your physical reactions to stressful
situations; then try to eliminate the triggers and control
those reactions.

• Tune in to your emotional response to stress and the
thoughts that accompany the feelings; then ask yourself if
these are the only appropriate thoughts you might have
about the situation.

• Experiment with biofeedback as a means of control.

• Take a course in cognitive behavioral therapy, then
apply its principles to stressful situations.

Modifying the adrenaline response isn't easy. Some people
may want to seek a counselor's help to do it. In many cases,
the adrenaline habit begins early, when a child doesn't feel
safe at home. The chemical changes that take place in the
brain of a child who lives in conditions of great physical or emotional stress are thought by some to be permanent. But the
brain is a very malleable organ, capable of adjustment and reor-
ganization even after severe physical injury. I see no reason
why a person for whom these words have personal significance
shouldn't make a special effort to overcome this problem.

Often people who survived traumatic childhoods want to
know if that is the cause of their fibromyalgia. Surely those
changes in brain chemistry make their contribution to the collection of symptoms, but just as surely many people who had
difficult childhoods don't develop FM. Those who do were
probably born with the predisposition to it and had no way to
avoid it. More important, even if you had the worst childhood
imaginable, how would it help you to assign blame to those
who caused your childhood stress? Would it make you feel any
better? Quite the opposite, it would probably make you think

there was no hope that you'd ever feel better than you do now. That kind of prediction certainly doesn't help improve the quality of your life. A far better response, if this applies to you, is to acknowledge what your childhood was like and then turn your attention to the things you will do to care for yourself and make your life better.

One of the many studies that have examined the characteristics of people who have fibromyalgia found that they are unusually sensitive to their environment.[12] The study also showed a connection between extreme sensitivity to outside stimuli and to pain. Since adrenaline is associated with hypervigilance, those of us with FM may do best in surroundings where noise and light levels are low. Of course, we can't always control the stimuli that surround us, but we can avoid situations that we know will be overstimulating, such as shopping malls and rock concerts. Doing so may also give us more control over our pain.

One of the basic drives of the human being is homeostasis—avoidance of change. To a great extent, our bodies are equipped to maintain equilibrium. For example, we have an internal control system that helps us adjust to changes in the temperature of the air around us, and the pupils of our eyes adjust in an effort to maintain a steady level of light reaching our brains. Broadly defined, stress is the result of anything that threatens homeostasis, whether of the body or mind. Hunger and cold cause stress. Looked at this way, some stress is inevitable. Your goal should be to manage unavoidable stress and to avoid stress that is unnecessary. As you strive to meet this goal, remember that stress does not cause fibromyalgia, but it does make it worse.

One interesting technique for reducing unnecessary stress is based on the hemisphere theory of the brain. According to this theory, which has plenty of support in clinical experience, the right half (or hemisphere) of the brain is devoted predominantly to creative and emotional activity, while the left hemisphere is the site of rational and analytical thinking.

You can take some pressure off the more-stressed hemisphere by switching activities. For example, if you find yourself depressed or emotionally agitated, reduce the pressure on your right brain by engaging the left hemisphere for a while: Write a letter, balance your checkbook, or organize your sock drawer. On the other hand, if you're feeling overburdened by demands on your time, give your left brain a rest by listening to music, singing, or drawing a picture, all right-brain activities.

• • Tips for Lifting Depression • •

• Think of all the things you would do for a dear friend who was sad or ill or both. Make a list. Check off the three to five things you'd be most likely to do if you could. Then do them for yourself, one each week, over the next three to five weeks.

• Each week add something to the end of the list. "Oh, no," you say, "I'll never get done!" Exactly. That's the point. There should never be an end to treating yourself as well as you'd treat a friend in need.

• Make a list of all the people you know who wouldn't be annoyed to hear your voice on the telephone. Call one each day, just to say hello. "I was thinking about you and just felt like saying hello" is a sufficient excuse for the call. Ask how the other person is feeling and what he or she is doing. If you're asked, say you're fine even if it's a lie (it won't be forever) and get back to talking about the person you called.

• For the next six months, accept all invitations that will allow you to get home before your normal bedtime. If invitations have stopped coming your way, invite a couple of people to visit and rejuvenate your social life.

• • • • • • • • • • • • • • • • • •

Cognitive Problems

When it comes to poor memory, we have plenty of company among NDAs. Let's start with the things we forget that NDAs forget, too. Names, for example. If you and I met at a support group meeting tonight and we happened to bump into each other sometime this week, your face would most likely look familiar to me and I might remember where we met, but I probably wouldn't remember your name. I expect you would say the same thing, but so would most people, regardless of their age and health status. Almost everyone you know fears running into someone whose name they forgot and who declares, "I'll bet you don't know who I am." I think that people who make such a remark deserve the answer they get. A simple reply is "You win that bet," accompanied by a big grin.

If you don't believe that NDAs have memory problems, consider this: There is a whole industry devoted to helping people overcome memory loss.

You can buy a sweatshirt emblazoned with the phrase "I suffer from CRS disease." (The first two words of the acronym CRS are *Can't remember*—I'm sure you can image what the third word is.) Stand-up comedians have dozens of jokes on memory failure. My favorite is the one about the man who has the Hereafter disease. "What's that?" he is asked. He explains, "When I go down to the cellar for something, I have to call up to my wife, 'Hey, honey, what am I here after?'"

If you wear glasses, you can buy a cord that will let them dangle from your neck when you take them off. You can buy an electronic device to put on your key chain so that when you can't find your keys you can clap your hands and the device will beep at you. If people weren't constantly misplacing their belongings, there would not be a market for such items. Books are written and seminars are given on improving your memory. If there weren't people willing to pay for all this help, an industry based on the fact that most people are forgetful would have no reason to exist. Surely not all of those eager learners have fibromyalgia.

However, the "brain fog" that people with FM speak of goes much deeper than remembering names or where you put your glasses. It has to do with not being able to access needed bits of information, although you know the information is there. It is about pulling facts together, holding enough pieces of information in your mind simultaneously so that you can figure something out. It is about being unable to focus on any one thing for more than a few minutes at a time. It has to do with difficulty in absorbing and recalling information, following directions, and estimating time and distance. For many people with fibromyalgia, the cognitive dysfunction that accompanies the disorder is both frightening and frustrating.

"More than anything else," says Frances, a disabled former software engineer in her forties, "it is this lack of cognitive ability that has made me unable to work, to make commitments or promise to meet deadlines, even on a volunteer level. I don't dare let people count on me, knowing that I may not be able to meet their expectations. If this part of my FM could be treated successfully, maybe I could be a real live contributing human being again."

Shirley, twenty-five, was a senior in high school when a diving accident provided the trigger for FM. She's married now and trying to help her husband, Jim, to build a home-based business. Jim says, "Shirley was practically a lightning calculator when we first met, but she has developed problems with attention span and her cognitive abilities deteriorated very noticeably in the first two years we were together." Shirley adds, "I can't remember from minute to minute what I am supposed to be doing with the company's paperwork. More than once I have lost every important paper for the business." Her guilt at being unable to hold a job or complete course work for an associate degree compounds her emotional pain and frustration.

Right now little is known about the causes of FM's cognitive disabilities. A number of researchers report seeing structural changes in brain scans done on some people who have fibromyalgia. People with FM have also been shown to have a decreased supply of oxygen in some parts of the brain. Cognitive problems can be induced even in NDAs by depriving them of sleep, so it's reasonable to assume that improving one's sleep would help relieve fibromyalgic difficulties in this area. Furthermore, mental confusion is listed as a possible side effect of most mood-altering and painkilling drugs. This is a good reason for using such drugs for as short a period as possible while searching for alternatives that don't compromise one's mental faculties. There's simply no way to determine which of these factors is most responsible for our frustrating mental lapses.

• • • • How to Cope with • • • • Cognitive Problems

• Learn to breathe more effectively. Most people with fibromyalgia are shallow breathers. While it isn't certain that the oxygen deprivation seen in some fibromyalgic brains causes cognitive problems, the assumption is reasonable, and deep breathing aids in relaxation and pain relief as well. A voice or speech teacher can help, and there are books that teach breathing.

• Consider trying the herb ginkgo biloba, available in health food stores. It has been shown to increase blood circulation to the brain and is used with some success to alleviate memory loss in Alzheimer's patients. People with high blood pressure should ask a health care practitioner first.

• Minimize mental "background noise." For many of us, our minds are constantly occupied by the thought that we won't be able to remember what we're being told. Thinking this way requires mental energy that could be used for remembering. Try to identify that thought and turn it off.

• Keep a calendar or agenda book. Use it to record everything: appointments, promises, medication changes, points you want to mention to your doctor at the next visit, even things you're sure you'll remember.

• Write everything on paper. Have a pencil and notepad in every room, preferably on a table next to a chair. When you answer the phone, pick up a pencil with the other hand. Write down the name of the person calling and a phrase describing the purpose of the call. Note any decisions or commitments made—both yours and the caller's. Be compulsive about transferring such notes to your calendar or agenda.

• Before placing a phone call, write down what you want to accomplish. Leave space for the information you obtain. If it's a business call, write the phone number and extension you are calling, the date, and the time. If you have to leave a message, make a note of it. If you make a connection, be sure to note the name of the person on the other end of the line. Don't be shy about asking how to spell names. Even Smith has multiple possible spellings.

• Keep a notebook in your car for storing written directions (or maps, if you can read them) of the route to places you'll visit more than once. If you write the directions on sticky-backed notes, you can stick them to your dashboard to consult while you're driving.

• Cultivate routines for tasks such as handling mail and paying bills—and stick to them.

• Clutter confuses. Schedule time on your calendar, as you would any appointment, to get organized. Work at it an hour or so at a time. Sort papers into four piles: Urgent and Important; Urgent but Not Important; Important but Not Urgent; Neither Urgent nor Important. *Urgent* means an action must be taken by a specific date; *important* means it must be done but there is no deadline. With luck, your "Neither Urgent nor Important" pile will be the largest. Throw it away. Tackle your "Urgent and Important" pile first, the "Important but Not Urgent" pile next. Seriously consider whether you can throw away some of the "Urgent but Not Important" pile.

• When a task looks gigantic, break it down into a series of smaller steps. List them in order, then do one at a time, checking each one off when it's completed.

• Use a multisensory approach to learning. Tape lectures for later review. Read aloud when you study. Highlight important passages. Write notes in book margins. Try to form mental images to reinforce what you want to remember.

• Use music and rhyme as memory aids. Try fitting your shopping list to a familiar tune, such as "Three Blind Mice" or "The Twelve Days of Christmas."

• Frustrating as it is, try to maintain a sense of humor about your cognitive problems. Explain the problem when it's appropriate; when it's not, laugh it off if you get caught. Remind yourself that everyone has memory lapses, even if they're not on the scale of ours. No one person will ever know all the times you've forgotten something. If you don't make an issue of it, others probably won't, either.

• Don't push. If you're having a bad day cognitively and can't simply take the day off work, devote your time to routine tasks that are minimally demanding but will give you a sense of accomplishment.

• Exercise your mind. Do puzzles, play games that challenge your logical and creative capacities, set memory tasks for yourself. For example, in an unfamiliar place try to make mental pictures of the way furniture and accessories are arranged, then see how much you can recall later.

Perhaps the best thing you can do to alleviate cognitive distress is to rethink your standards. You're a worthwhile person because of who you are, not what you do.

• • • • • • • • • • • • • • • • • • •

Energy Conservation

Simply having enough energy to get through the day is a major issue for many people who have fibromyalgia. It's more than just not getting enough sleep, although that is part of the problem. But there is evidence that our bodies don't make efficient use of the food we eat, either because of faulty metabolism or because we don't absorb nutrients from our food effectively. Energy is like money; if you don't have enough, you have to learn to use it wisely, conserving it as much as possible so it will be there when you need it. This section suggests ways to do that.

• • Tips for Conserving Energy • •

• Budget your energy as you do your money. Plan your day; don't just let it happen.

• Set priorities. Try to strike a balance between what you must do and what you want to do. Continually ask yourself, "Is this task necessary?"

• Go easy on yourself. Learn to say no. Say "That won't be possible" instead of "I can't."

• Notice at what time of day you feel your best, and take advantage of that time to do the most demanding things on your list.

• Remember the motto "Divide and conquer." When you're facing a major task, break it down into smaller tasks and tackle one at a time.

• Recognize that you can't do everything. If you live with other people, delegate some essential chores.

• Negotiate with the people around you. Take on tasks you can do more easily and trade away those that are most difficult. (Running the vacuum cleaner tops the tough-job list of most people with fibromyalgia.)

• Make daily and weekly "to-do" lists so that you don't have to waste mental energy reminding yourself of everything you have to do. Check items off as you finish them to boost your sense of accomplishment.

• Avoid rushing. Nothing that is done in a hurry is done well.

• Rest frequently and stop before you become exhausted.

• Watch what you eat (see the next chapter, on nutrition). Food is fuel. Give yourself the best fuel you can.

• • • • • • • • • • • • • • • • • • •

If you're really interested in this subject, I have a project for you. It should be done for a few minutes a day over several days, rather than all at once. That way, your subconscious has plenty of time to think about things. Thoughts will come to you at odd moments; write them down. The project involves making a detailed analysis of your activities:

• List the roles you play. Here are some suggestions: parent; daughter/son; husband/wife; grandparent; employee/employer; friend; neighbor; sister/brother; niece/ nephew; cousin; aunt/uncle; church member; student/ teacher; patient; nurse; homeowner; landlord; volunteer; adviser; mentor; cook; chauffeur; house cleaner; shopper; bookkeeper; landscaper. Add more as you think of them.

• Pick one of these roles that you find difficult but necessary or desirable.

• List the activities required of you in this role.

• Choose one of the activities on this list that you find difficult, stressful, or fatiguing.

• Analyze that activity, jotting down thoughts about how to make it less stressful or tiring. For each activity, ask yourself:
  • Can you choose a different time of day to do it?
  • Do you have the proper equipment and supplies?
  • Does the position of your body when you do it drain your energy? Cause pain?
  • Can you break the activity down into steps? Eliminate some steps? Get help?
  • Is there adaptive equipment that you can use for this activity?

Don't overlook the need to conserve mental energy. This means, among other things, avoiding negative thoughts and not using your mind to worry about things that aren't worth the worry. Your brain accounts for no more than 2 percent of your body weight, but it consumes 20 percent of all the energy you get from your food. In other words, your brain burns up ten times as much energy, pound for pound, as the rest of your body.[13] Much of this energy is consumed in running the rest of your body, keeping you breathing, making your heart beat, and so forth. But you control the portion that is used for thought— don't waste it needlessly.

8

Fight Back with Good Nutrition

When I was in fourth grade, my teacher, Miss Kirwin, dealt with health education as follows: She would glare at the class, shake a finger at her students, and proclaim, "You *are* what you eat!" We children, an irreverent bunch of nine-year-olds, thought that was hilarious. We'd run around the lunchroom waving a hot dog on a roll, giggling, and declare, "Today I am a hot dog." But now I know that Miss Kirwin was right. There is no condition of the human body that cannot be made worse by faulty nutrition, so it must follow that one's physical condition can be improved by excellent nutrition. What we ingest has a direct effect on the body's building blocks. Bones, muscles, nerves, bodily fluids, chemicals—where can they come from if not from our food?

As important as nutrition is to our health, a survey by the National Research Council found that barely one quarter of medical schools in the United States require students to take even one course in nutrition.[14] No wonder that many doctors think nutrition is of minor importance. This is one of the failures of modern Western medicine. Although some medical schools are beginning to recognize the importance of nutrition in the curriculum, few physicians in practice today have more than a rudimentary understanding of the relationship between their patients' health and dietary intake. Thus, many doctors tell their patients that if they eat a balanced diet there is no need for supplementary vitamins. However, if pressed to define a balanced diet, these doctors will either shrug or point to a pyramid chart on the wall that specifies certain food groups and a certain number of servings of each.

Few doctors—and only a small percentage of the general population—know that the nutritional value of today's commercially processed food is inferior to that of food available in the past. Food used to be grown in soil that was fertilized with natural substances (that is, decomposed organic wastes). The switch to artificial petrochemical fertilizers has resulted, over time, in such a severe depletion of the world's soils that food harvested today is already deficient in nutrients. Whereas food was consumed locally and soon after harvest in the past, sophisticated shipping and storage techniques are now used with commercially produced food. But these techniques are rarely designed to preserve whatever nutrients are left in the food. So even though we may feed ourselves and our families the best food we can provide, the likelihood is still strong that we will not be nourished sufficiently for robust good health.

Also bear in mind that several studies have shown that people with FM absorb and metabolize nutrients inefficiently. According to other studies, people who suffer from malnutrition at *any* time in their lives will subsequently have an abnormally high need for certain nutrients. (The first study of this sort dealt with concentration camp survivors, who required massive doses of B vitamins for the rest of their lives.) This all points to the need of people with FM to supplement their diets with vitamins and minerals that are present in insufficient quantities in the food they eat.

Although many studies have been done, many more should be done, but they are not being undertaken because of economics and the profit motive. There is little or no profit in funding studies that show that people can make themselves feel better, if not entirely well, by improving their nutritional intake. It is up to us as people with FM, people who want to feel well and live full lives, to take care of ourselves. We can use doctors as sources of some information and advice, in addition to educating ourselves and using our own common sense and experience. Don't reject doctors because they don't know everything we'd like them to know about nutrition; nor should we defer to their lack of knowledge on the subject.

You Are What You Eat

There's not enough room in this book to tell you all you should know about nutrition, but you would do yourself (and your family) an enormous favor by learning what constitutes a superior diet and then planning your meals accordingly. The "Resources" section lists some recommended books on nutrition.

Conventional wisdom holds to three basic principles of good nutrition:

- About 60 to 65 percent of your daily food intake (in terms of calories, not ounces or grams) should consist of complex carbohydrates: fresh fruits and vegetables, grains, pasta, potatoes.

- No more than 25 percent of your daily intake should be made up of fats: butter, cheese, nuts, oils primarily.

- The remaining 15 to 20 percent of your diet should consist of proteins: fish, poultry, lean meat (be sure to consider the fat content of meat), beans.

Some people, however, do not thrive on this diet. In fact, a diet this high in carbohydrates causes some people to experience intestinal gas and bloating and makes others gain weight. Recent research suggests that people with certain ethnic backgrounds and body types do better on a diet that contains a

higher proportion of proteins and fats and very few carbohydrates. If you're following the conventional dietary guidelines
and wonder if a change might help you to feel better, an easy
and harmless way to experiment is to follow for two or three
weeks a yeast elimination diet in one of the books on yeast
overgrowth listed in the "Resources" section. If you don't feel
much better, and possibly slimmer, after that, a high-protein
diet is probably not for you.

Regardless of the proportion of proteins, carbohydrates, and
fats in your diet, as much as possible you should avoid caffeine,
refined sugar, alcohol, and artificial sweeteners. This is true for
everyone, but especially for people with fibromyalgia.

Many, if not most, people with fibromyalgia have a tendency
toward reactive hypoglycemia. In this condition, the pancreas
overreacts to the presence of glucose (derived from carbohydrates), producing too much of the hormone insulin, which facilitates its use in the body for energy or stores it for later use.
When a person eats refined sugar—white sugar and any of the
foodstuffs ending in *-ose* (sucrose, dextrose, fructose, for example)—this process takes place as soon as the sugar-containing
food reaches the stomach. With complex, unrefined sugars, it
takes place later in the small intestine.

The sudden rush of simple sugars from the stomach into the
bloodstream triggers a rush of insulin, which causes the level
of glucose (digested sugar) in the blood to drop rapidly. Sens-
ing an emergency in the bloodstream, the adrenal glands put
out adrenaline to draw glucose from the liver and return the
blood sugar to its proper level. The low-blood-sugar phase of
reactive hypoglycemia is responsible for symptoms such as
sleepiness, fatigue, headache, and sometimes even fainting.
The release of adrenaline triggers in some people the same
symptoms they would experience if they were in danger: rapid
heartbeat, racing pulse, and the feeling of panic. People who
experience this reaction in daytime call it a panic attack; at
night the same phenomenon is usually interpreted as a nightmare.

Reactive hypoglycemia, the sudden drop in blood sugar in reaction to an incoming flood of sugar and the overreaction of the pancreas and adrenal glands in trying to maintain the body's normal blood sugar level, is very common among people who have fibromyalgia.

Vitamin Supplements

Probably everyone needs supplementary vitamins to make up for the nutrients missing in the soil, and for those lost during transit and storage of produce on its way to the market. People with FM have even greater nutritional needs than most people. Many of us meet those needs with vitamin and mineral supplements. Which specific supplements you need and in what quantities is a highly individual matter. Some health care practitioners can perform blood tests to determine the levels of vitamins and minerals in your body, and this is an ideal way to arrive at your supplement plan. If that's not possible for you, you can read about the various vitamins and minerals and experiment for yourself with supplements, deciding which to try according to the symptoms listed for various deficiencies. The primary danger in the latter approach is that you may waste money on substances you don't really need. If you're taking a multivitamin now, you're probably already doing that. Multiple vitamin preparations are formulated to suit some mythical average person, and you can bet that's a healthy and active young man, not you. Your needs are unique.

You would have to spend a great deal of money and take a huge number of vitamin pills to overdose on the water-soluble vitamins: the B-complex vitamins and C. This is because these vitamins dissolve in water and wash out of your body in your urine, rather than being stored in your tissues. (Vitamin B_{12} is the exception; it is capable of being stored in the liver.) The oil-soluble vitamins—A, D, and E—are dissolved by fats, which is why you should never strive to eliminate fats entirely from you diet. Vitamins A, D, and E are stored in your liver and body fat; it *is* possible to take too much of any of them. Table 8-1 lists vitamins, their major functions, and suggested daily doses of each. Maximum safe doses of the fat-soluble vitamins are also given. Water-soluble vitamins are measured in milligrams (mg) or micrograms (mcg). One milligram is 1/1,000th of a gram; one microgram is 1/1,000th of a milligram. Fat-soluble vitamins are measured in International Units (IU).

Remember that these dosage suggestions are for people of normal health. If you choose to experiment with vitamins, you should find your own optimal level by starting below the suggested dose in table 8-1 and working up gradually. By paying attention to how you feel each day, you will discover the best doses for yourself. It may take a few weeks to see results, so be patient and attentive.

If necessary, you can make a couple of substitutions in the accompanying table. Some people experience facial flushing when they take vitamin B₃ (niacin) in large doses. An alternative is niacinamide, which does not have this effect. However, niacinamide does not have the same cardiovascular benefits as niacin. Another acceptable substitution is beta-carotene for vitamin A. Beta-carotene is a precursor to vitamin A—that is, it turns into vitamin A in the body—but it only makes as much vitamin A as the body needs. Even if you were to take enough beta-carotene to turn your complexion orange (the sign of a toxic vitamin A overdose), you would not experience toxicity. Suggested daily dose is 15 IU of beta-carotene, which equals 25,500 IU of vitamin A. This does not approach toxic levels, because beta-carotene not used for vitamin A has other purposes. Working in concert with vitamins C and E, beta-carotene is a powerful antioxidant, helping to prevent the formation of malignant cancer cells.

Did you know that vitamin D is the only vitamin that you can obtain directly from the environment as well as from food? It is made when the sun's ultraviolet rays interact with the oils

Table 8-1: Guide to Vitamin Supplements

Vitamin	Function	Suggested Daily Dose	Toxicity Warning
A	Strengthens skin, vision, bones, nails, hair, resistance to viral infections.	4,000–5,000 IU	25,000 IU
B$_1$ (Thiamine)	Converts carbohydrates into energy; serves as mild diuretic; helps body deal with stress.	100 mg	
B$_2$ (Riboflavin)	Converts proteins, fats into energy; maintains body's tissues; helps body deal with stress.	50 mg	
B$_3$ (Niacin)	Promotes fat synthesis, protein metabolism; helps body deal with stress; promotes cardiovascular health.	50 mg	
B$_5$ (Pantothenic Acid)	Supports general nutrient metabolism, especially amino acids; participates in manufacture of many hormones; helps in nerve regulation.	200 mg	
B$_6$ (Pyridoxine)	Strenghens immune system; plays role in nerve impulse transmission; deficiency can cause depression, carpal tunnel syndrome.	150 mg	6 grams (6,000 mg)
B$_{12}$ (Cobalamin)	Aids nervous system, production of hemoglobin in blood; can help treat memory loss, depression, insomnia.	100 mcg	

Table 8-1 (continued)

Vitamin	Function	Suggested Daily Dose	Toxicity Warning
Folate (*Folic Acid*)	Helps in formation of hemoglobin in blood.	400 mcg	
Biotin	Acts in metabolism of nutrients in foods; helps maintain healthy skin.	50 mcg	
Inositol	Reduces LDL ("bad") cholesterol; aids sleep; reduces anxiety.	200 mg	
C (*Ascorbic Acid*)	Fortifies immune system; helps reduce effects of physical and psychological stress; may reduce elevated cholesterol.	2 grams (2,000 mg)	10 grams (10,000 mg)
D	Promotes bone, tooth health; regulates blood calcium level, absorption and distribution of digested calcium.	200 IU (more during dark winter months)	1,000 IU
E	Promotes blood health, aids circulation.	400 IU	1,200 IU

Note: Suggested doses and toxicity warnings are based on information in *How to Be Your Own Nutritionist*, by Stuart M. Berger M.D. (New York: Avon Books, 1987) and *Earl Mindell's Vitamin Bible*, by Earl Mindell, Ph.D., R.Ph. (New York: Warner Books, 1991).

on your skin and is absorbed into your body through your pores. There is evidence of a relationship between seasonal affective disorder (SAD) and a deficiency in vitamin D. People who suffer from winter depression might well consider supplementing with vitamin D. Cod liver oil, available in capsules, is a good natural source of vitamin D as well as vitamin A.

Vitamin K, not listed in the table, is the source of the blood-clotting substance prothrombin, which prevents excessive blood flow. Vitamin K is plentiful in a wide variety of common foods. It is also manufactured by a species of bacteria that lives in our intestines. There is no need to supplement vitamin K unless you have been told to do so by a physician.

Special Note: If you have diabetes, an autoimmune disease such as multiple sclerosis, and/or if you are undergoing chemotherapy, do not take vitamin supplements without first consulting a doctor or nutritionist with knowledge and experience in this area. (Fibromyalgia is not an autoimmune disease.)

Mineral Supplements

Minerals come to us from our food and, in some localities, from drinking water. The mineral content of fruits and vegetables depends heavily on where they are grown. Unlike vitamins, minerals are not likely to deteriorate during shipping and storage, nor are they depleted by chemical fertilizers. For most people, a single multimineral supplement pill a day is ample.

The minerals most important to people who have fibromyalgia are calcium and magnesium. Calcium is important to the functioning of the cardiovascular system. It also helps conduct nerve impulses, participates in the contraction of muscles, and helps in the coagulation of blood at the site of a wound. Its most crucial function, however, is in the formation of bones and teeth. Women who have had their ovaries removed and those who are past menopause are at risk of osteoporosis, or brittle bone disease, brought on by a lack of calcium. Vitamins C and D are required for the absorption of calcium to occur. For men and premenopausal women, a daily dose of 1,000 mg of calcium is sufficient. After the onset of menopause the recommended dose is 1,500 mg. Calcium comes in four forms: carbonate, phosphate, gluconate, and lactate. Calcium carbonate is the best in terms of availability to the body. It is usually also the least expensive.

If you are taking calcium, you should balance it with magnesium. Calcium tends to be constipating; magnesium has the opposite, laxative, effect. Magnesium facilitates the work of calcium in your body. It collaborates with some 300 enzymes in your body that control all kinds of vital life processes. It helps lower blood pressure and, most important to people who have fibromyalgia, it helps prevent muscle spasms. People with restless or jerky legs often find it helpful. The optimal ratio of calcium to magnesium is 1.5:1 or 2:1—for example, 1,500 mg of calcium and 750 to 1,000 mg of magnesium. Calcium-magnesium combination tablets are easy to find in the vitamin section of your pharmacy, supermarket, or health food store.

Amino Acids

Amino acids derived from our food are the building blocks from which proteins are made. They also provide the raw materials for some of the neurochemicals we have in insufficient quantities. Blood tests reveal that many people with FM are deficient in amino acids, which may help explain such problems as insomnia, depression, and lack of energy. It seems reasonable that amino acid supplements may help us feel better. The material that follows will help you decide whether this is an avenue worth exploring further. For more information on the therapeutic use of amino acids, consult the books listed in the "Resources" section and a knowledgeable practitioner.

There are nine essential amino acids. *Essential* in this context means not only that they are necessary to the functioning of the human body, but also that your body is unable to create them in adequate amounts from other raw materials. They are used both to form protein cells and to create the fifteen nonessential amino acids that your body can synthesize. In other words, "nonessential" amino acids, while necessary to sustain life, are not needed as raw materials for other amino acids. Even some of these, however, can be "essential" in some individuals, particularly in children and the elderly.

The essential amino acids, which you must get from food or supplementary sources, are histidine, methionine, tryptophan, isoleucine, lysine, threonine, leucine, phenylalanine, and valine. Every amino acid comes in two forms, a "left-handed" or L form and a "right-handed" or D form. They are as alike and as different as your left and right hands. Like your hands, unless you are truly ambidextrous, they have somewhat different capabilities. In the discussion that follows, I will omit the prefix *L,* but you may assume that I am talking about the left-handed form unless I specify otherwise. These essential amino acids contain the raw materials for the rest of the amino family: cysteine, cystine, tyrosine, arginine, alanine, glutamic acid, proline, hydroxyproline, glutamine, histidine, aspartic acid, glycine, serine, asparagine, and carnitine.

Individuals vary enormously in their amino acid requirements, and the requirements of a single individual can vary widely depending on a variety of factors: stress, exercise level, current health status, trauma, temperature extremes, the presence of toxic substances in the environment (for example, atmospheric pollution) and in the diet (such as alcohol and caffeine), and the use of therapeutic or recreational drugs. Several experiments have discovered variations in amino acid requirements between individuals ranging from three- to ninefold, with an average difference of a factor of five.[15] This is important information; it shows just how important it is for each person to be treated individually. Using someone else's results to determine your own needs can cause an imbalance in your own system. However, lest I overstate the case, let me remind you that your body's own internal regulating mechanisms, always striving toward homeostasis, provide a potent safety valve. I mean to caution you, not to frighten you.

First on the list of amino acids that should interest people with fibromyalgia, as well as those who suffer from depression and chronic pain, is tryptophan. It is present in meat and dairy products primarily, although smaller amounts are found in many other foods. A pound (453 grams) of roast beef contains 1,154 mg of tryptophan; a pound of roast lamb contains 1,525 mg. Since 1,500 to 2,000 mg of tryptophan is the dose many people find useful as an aid to sleep, you can see that it's not reasonable to expect food alone to provide you with a good night's sleep, although the tryptophan in turkey may be largely responsible for the nap we take after our Thanksgiving Day dinner.

Tryptophan can be measured in the blood, and many people with fibromyalgia have been found to have subnormal levels of serum tryptophan. This finding may provide a clue to the insomnia we experience, and may also explain depression in some people. Tryptophan, working with a couple of enzymes and vitamin B_6, acts in the brain to create serotonin (whose chemical name is 5-HT), which is involved with sleep, mood, and pain perception. In an intermediate step, before it becomes serotonin, tryptophan breaks down into two compounds: kynurenine and 5-hydroxytryptophan (5-HTP). Kynurenine's function has no bearing on this discussion, but 5-HTP is the direct precursor of serotonin. One current theory holds that people who have fibromyalgia do not break tryptophan down efficiently, perhaps because they don't absorb it well, or because they lack the necessary enzymes. 5-HTP, therefore, may provide a solution to the tryptophan problem in certain cases.

Some people who have taken tryptophan as a supplement have found it quite useful in alleviating insomnia. I once surveyed people discussing fibromyalgia on the Internet, specifically those who had taken tryptophan before a contaminated batch led to its removal from the market. I asked these individuals whether they found it useful and would take it again if they could. Of nearly ninety people who responded, all but one said they did, and they would. Tryptophan is once again available, most commonly from a compounding pharmacy, and requires a prescription (see "Resources"); its breakdown product, 5-HTP, is similarly available and may for some be a more efficient way of elevating levels of serotonin. Like everything else, however, some people find it useless. People who are taking a drug that blocks the reabsorption of serotonin at the receptor site (known as a specific serotonin reuptake inhibitor, or SSRI, such as Wellbutrin, Zoloft, or Luvox) should not take tryptophan or 5-HTP lest they overload their systems with serotonin. Also, women who are pregnant and those taking an MAO inhibitor such as Marplan, Nardil, or Parnate should not consider tryptophan.

Phenylalanine is another essential amino acid that some will want to explore, but not if they are taking an MAO inhibitor. (People who have phenylketonuria, a rare metabolic disorder that makes them unable to break down phenylalanine, must also avoid it. It is hardly possible to reach adulthood without knowing if you have this disorder.) Phenylalanine converts to another amino acid, tyrosine, and from there to the neurotransmitter dopamine, and eventually to the adrenal hormones norepinephrine and epinephrine (also known as adrenaline). Some people find phenylalanine beneficial in terms of energy and helpful in overcoming the effects of adrenal inadequacy. Those who want to shorten the metabolic cycle, as well as those deficient in the enzyme that converts phenylalanine to tyrosine, might think about taking tyrosine instead. I have tried both, at 500 mg each (not at the same time), and decided to stay with tyrosine. An interesting side effect of taking tyrosine (and phenylalanine before it) is that I sweat when I exercise, whereas before I simply turned beet red, my skin got hot, and I looked as if I was on the verge of a stroke.

A mixture of the D and L forms of phenylalanine, called D-L-phenylalanine or DLPA, can be useful for pain relief. It takes between one and four weeks to reach optimum benefit, and researchers have found that after it is discontinued, its effects last for up to a month. DLPA is readily available in health food stores. No adverse effects have been reported, and its effects do not seem to diminish with use. DLPA's action is to increase the activity of endorphins, the brain's natural answer to morphine. The usual daily dosage is two 375 mg tablets taken at least a half hour before each meal, for a total of six tablets. If there is no improvement within three weeks, the dosage may be doubled. If there is still no response after a week or so, the product should be discontinued. The failure rate is reported to be between 5 and 15 percent.[16]

One of the functions of the essential amino acid arginine is to stimulate the pituitary gland's production of growth hormone. It is also said to aid in glucose (sugar) tolerance and improve fertility. However, arginine definitely has its downside. It stimulates the growth of the herpes virus. People who tend to get herpes simplex cold sores or have genital herpes should steer clear of arginine and arginine-rich foods, including corn, peanuts, chocolate, and edible seeds. Herpes zoster, the virus that causes shingles in one who has had chicken pox—no matter how many years before—has been known to flare up in people taking arginine. An antidote for this is the essential amino acid lysine, which people plagued with herpes might also consider taking independently, since it has been shown to halt the development of that virus. Because most people with fibromyalgia are deficient in growth hormone, it might be worthwhile to watch for reports on clinical trials of arginine. For now, I wouldn't advise trying it without the support of an experienced clinician.

Yeast Overgrowth: Is There a Connection?

Candida albicans is a single-celled yeastlike plant that is part of the normal population of the human gut. Under normal circumstances it lives peacefully within us. It reproduces by putting out buds, which is what makes it like yeast. One *Candida* cell can reproduce billions of times. Friendly (to us) intestinal bacteria, various enzymes, and some hormones normally prevent a population explosion of *C. albicans* organisms, and its presence in our bodies is of no consequence. Some events in our lives can provide the proper conditions for *Candida* to flourish. Among those events are taking antibiotics, corticosteroids, or oral contraceptives. A weakened immune system can permit *Candida* to proliferate, as can various nutritional deficiencies.

Why am I telling you this? Because while I was writing this book I found it necessary to start doing research on *Candida*— for highly personal reasons. I had been losing my hearing at a rate that increasing age could not explain; nor could the otologist I consulted suggest any other possibility once he had ruled out autoimmune inner ear disease. Frightened at the thought of impending deafness, I did what I always do when something threatens me: I set out to learn everything I could about it. I found reference to the treatment of hearing loss and oral nystatin, a bacterium commonly used to treat yeast infections.[18] I got my doctor to prescribe it for me, and it stopped the progressive hearing loss for as long as I took it. (This story is not over yet; the hearing loss resumed, so I'm taking nystatin again.)

Recently, events conspired to weaken my normally strong immune system, and I found myself overrun by yeast. Again, I turned to research and discovered a long list of symptoms attributed to yeast infestation that sound very much like what we experience with fibromyalgia. I'm not suggesting that fibromyalgia is caused by yeast, but it's clear to me that many symptoms associated with FM can be made worse by yeast overgrowth. Among the symptoms that caught my attention are:

- low-grade fever
- night sweats
- shortness of breath on minor exertion
- blurred vision
- persistent and severe headaches

- depression
- cognitive difficulty, attention deficit disorder
- numbness and tingling
- dry eyes
- abnormal sensitivity to light
- tinnitus (ringing in the ears)
- hearing loss
- vertigo
- edema (swelling of tissues)
- frequent/urgent urination
- vaginitis
- multiple allergies and chemical sensitivities
- cravings for carbohydrates, including sugar
- feeling particularly ill on days when humidity is high.

I also learned that yeast overgrowth can interfere with absorption of nutrients in the gut, which is where we absorb most of the beneficial components of the food we eat.[19] This could—I'm not saying it does, only that it might—explain why some people with fibromyalgia are unable to get the benefit of tryptophan in the foods they eat. It might have a great deal to do with hormone imbalances in general.

To stave off yeast proliferation, I am presently doing the following: I eat a diet consisting only of proteins and vegetables. This diet deprives my yeasts of the sugars they need to grow and reproduce. I'm seeing great results and will soon start adding carbohydrates gradually (but never again refined sugars and possibly not fruit juices). I have added to my dietary supplements acidophilus (a bacterium friendly to us but death to yeasts), caprylic acid (an essential fatty acid that yeast hates), and deodorized garlic (real garlic is fine, but it makes you stinky).

Some doctors scoff at this regimen, so don't be surprised if you mention it to your doctor and are told to forget it. There is plenty of research on the behavior of yeast in diabetics, on people who have HIV disease or AIDS, and some on yeast in people whose immune systems have been compromised by chemotherapy for cancer or by long courses of steroids, but little is to be found on yeast in otherwise healthy individuals. I'm sure this will not be true for much longer.

I'll continue learning what I can and will post my findings on my World Wide Web site (see "Resources," where I've also listed some books on the subject).

Your Responsibilities and Risks

The message to take away from this chapter is that there are now, and will be increasingly in the future, nutrients that can help us. (Considerable research is under way on a class of nutrients known as essential fatty acids, but I've seen nothing yet worth acting on.) I believe that nutritional therapies will eventually emerge as the first line of defense against the effects of fibromyalgia. At a minimum, you owe it to yourself and those you care about to provide as wholesome and nourishing a diet as possible, avoiding fast foods (because they are full of fats and needless salt), snack foods (for the same reason), and sweets (for their effect on blood sugar levels and the release of adrenaline). NDAs may be able to get by with poor nutrition; people with fibromyalgia certainly cannot.

Is there a risk in experimenting with vitamin supplements and amino acids? Of course there is. Nothing is without risk: Walking down a flight of stairs, eating a hamburger, or driving a car carries some risk. So does taking vitamins, minerals, amino acids, herbs—or prescription medicines. In any given year, approximately 63,000 Americans die from taking prescription drugs as their doctors prescribed them. That's about three times the number of people who die from intentional homicide.[17] If anything near that number of people died, or even became ill, from taking nutritional supplements, you can be sure the U.S. government would ban them from the market-place. My experience in talking with hundreds of people who have fibromyalgia is that those who are experiencing the best quality in their lives used heavy-duty painkillers and/or psychoactive drugs only long enough to get themselves back to the point where they could think rationally about their condition. Then they mapped out a strategy that involves minimizing drug intake, engaging in exercise, and practicing the best possible nutrition, supplementation, and sleep hygiene.

9

Exercise to Combat Depression and Pain

Cindy was a happy, healthy twenty-four-year-old when injuries resulting from an automobile accident forced her to stay in bed for a long period of recuperation. Her wounds healed, but she never recovered. Symptoms of fibromyalgia (a term she didn't even know) replaced those of her injuries. She couldn't get out of bed; the pain was too severe.

Cindy was thirty and bedridden for six years when I first heard from her by telephone. She had seen many doctors, several of whom had suggested psychiatric hospitalization and none of whom had helped her. She wanted to know if I thought she had FM. I assisted her in finding a doctor familiar with fibromyalgia, but it took a lot of encouragement from her friends to get her to make an appointment because she feared yet another disappointment. Also, since she could not sit for more than a few minutes at a time, the logistics of getting her to her appointment were quite complicated. The doctor made the diagnosis of fibromyalgia. She prescribed a low dose of an antidepressant and something for pain relief to get Cindy out of the crisis she was in. A couple of weeks passed before Cindy saw any improvement, during which time she relied heavily on the support system she had assembled for herself. Gradually, her sleep improved and her pain became manageable, but she was still too weak to get out of bed except for an occasional trip to the bathroom and a shower in the morning.

Cindy and I began to talk about ways to build her endurance. Walking seemed impossible to her, let alone a routine of stretching and strengthening exercises, but I knew that without exercise she would never regain her ability to function independently. I suggested that she double the amount of exercise she was currently getting by walking to and from the bathroom twice every time she went there. She thought she could do that and agreed to try. I told her that when the two trips became easy, as I assured her they would, she should add a third and keep increasing the number of trips until she could walk the length of her apartment and back without fatigue.

A month later Cindy called to say that she had been outside for a five-minute walk for the first time in six years. She put film in her camera and resumed her hobby of photography. Cindy was on her way, we both agreed. By this time Cindy was convinced that the only way to regain as much of her former strength as possible was to keep moving. I suggested that she approach her recovery as though it were her full-time job, walking as much as she could without fatigue and learning everything she could during the hours she was in bed about exercise, pain management, and nutrition as they relate to FM. Eight months after her diagnosis Cindy sent me a Christmas card on which she wrote: "I am up about three hours a day now. I feel that the progress is slow, but my doctor is *impressed!* You were right. I've had to make my recovery a full-time job, but it's worth it."

I tell Cindy's story as an example of how even small efforts add up to bring improvement. Many of us are caught up in the modern quest for a quick fix, a pill that will make everything better right away. But with fibromyalgia, there is no such thing, and hoping that a quick cure will appear detracts from the possibility of helping ourselves achieve a better quality of life. Even the best doctors can help only so much; the rest is up to us. We all have work to do, constantly, not only on our physical beings but also on our minds.

The Benefits of Exercise

It is almost a sure thing that you will feel better if you exercise regularly. I get into trouble with someone every time I say this in a presentation to a support group. The only reason I say "almost" is that I've known two people out of the hundreds with whom I've discussed exercise who say they were in top aerobic shape when FM struck, and that exercise neither prevented their getting sick nor helped them get well. Most people agree that exercise is crucial to their well-being.

A few are absolutely convinced that they don't dare try to exercise, so they never find out whether it would help them. I understand this group very well. In fact, I used to feel the same way. For most of my adult life until early 1990, I didn't move if I didn't have to. If I could get someone to climb stairs for me when I needed something that was on another floor in the house, I did. If I could get someone to bend over and pick things up for me when I dropped them, I did. I didn't walk if I could avoid it, I didn't stand if I could sit, and I didn't sit if I could lie down—this, believe it or not, on a doctor's advice. In 1989 I developed sciatic pain worse than any pain I'd ever experienced—including unmedicated childbirth—and landed in bed (again at a doctor's suggestion) for the better part of six months. By the time I was finished with my stint in bed, my muscles were so weak that I knew I had to try some sort of exercise if I was to regain any strength.

I bought a book on stretching that my physical therapist had recommended, but at first I did only those stretches I could do in bed, because I feared if I got down on the floor I'd never be able to get up again. Over the next year I learned to stretch and then to do some gentle strengthening exercises. It has been my experience that every time I stop exercising, either by choice or by necessity, it takes me somewhat longer than the last time to regain what I've lost. It took me most of 1990 to regain what little flexibility and strength I had before my time in bed.

I read about the benefits of aerobic exercise and wanted to

try it. But I live in a very hilly area where temperatures can range from minus twenty degrees Fahrenheit in the wintertime to ninety-five degrees in the summer. I could readily imagine all the excuses I'd be able to find to avoid walking outside: bad weather, sore knees, not enough time, and so forth. Instead, I bought a stationary bicycle, the kind with a resistance adjustment so that you can work hard or with less intensity, depending on your level of fitness and how you feel. When I first got on that bike, with resistance set to zero so the wheels turned freely, I knew I'd made a big mistake. By the time the timer got to 3½ minutes, I thought I was going to die. I was panting, my legs were shaking, and I was starting to feel nauseated. Stubborn as I was, and unwilling to waste the money I'd spent on the bike, I got back on the next morning, this time for only three minutes. I had bone-deep aches in my legs, but I was feeling panicky about the prospect of being an invalid for the rest of my life, so I tried to ignore the pain and, to my surprise, it eased up a bit soon after I started cycling. As the week went on, I found myself hurting less and less each day. Even more important, my normally somewhat-depressed mood was improving. I rode that bike before breakfast for three minutes, then four, then five—increasing a minute at a time when the previous level of exercise began to seem easy. Although I'm sure I had fibromyalgia in those days, it would be three more years before I first heard the word, on the day I got my diagnosis.

During those three years I worked up to a twenty-minute stationary bike ride at moderate resistance. I also backslid from time to time; I'd find some good and pressing reason to stop biking. Invariably, by the time I'd been off my exercise routine for three weeks, my feeling of depression was back. It became clear to me that this depression was of chemical origin—there was nothing in my life to justify being sad, let alone depressed. It eventually dawned on me that there was some relationship between my lack of exercise and my mood. I decided I was addicted to bicycling.

I rode that stationary bike most days for six years until, in the summer of 1996, the electronic component that set the resistance and counted off the minutes broke. I called the manufacturer to order a new part and kept riding, without resistance, because it was all I could think of to do. By that time I had discovered 5-HTP and was sleeping pretty well. My pain level was down to about a three on a ten-point scale. But within three weeks of no-resistance exercising while I waited for the part to arrive, I found I was getting depressed and achy again. And this time I was scared, because I had a business trip coming up—an important conference I couldn't afford to miss.

I dragged myself to the conference. As soon as I got settled in the hotel room, I put on my sweats, headed for the exercise room, and got on a stationary bike. I made it to twenty minutes, and by the time I was walking back to my room I could feel my mood lifting and my pain receding. If I had any lingering doubt about the importance of exercise in my life, I became a true believer at that point.

When I got home from that trip—in much better shape than when I left, to my surprise—I learned that the manufacturer couldn't supply the replacement part. I have now replaced the stationary bike with a cross-trainer, and I've been exercising every day but Sunday (so it doesn't feel quite like a life sentence) ever since. Exercise can be boring, but the difference in how I feel after I'm done and for the rest of the day is so amazing that I'd be really stupid to stop.

The fact that aerobic exercise is repetitive may hold the key to its effectiveness in lessening the pain and fatigue of fibromyalgia. Low-level, monotonous stimulation of the portion of the brain called the hypothalamus causes it to produce a brain chemical known as endorphins.[20] Endorphins are the brain's own natural painkillers. Their chemical signature is almost identical to that of opium and its derivative, morphine. Endorphins work in the same way that opiate drugs do, by damping down the pathways in the nervous system that respond to pain signals. While substance P, the brain's chemical pain messenger, travels straight up the spinal column to the brain, endorphins are released into the bloodstream, making their pain relief longer lasting than the pain signal itself. A good workout can produce enough endorphins to last twenty-four hours or more.

Not only do endorphins relieve pain, but they also enhance the production of serotonin, which probably explains why people who exercise regularly often become moody and edgy when they stop. In addition, while we produce 80 percent of our growth hormone during deep sleep, the other 20 percent comes about as the result of vigorous exercise. These are the arguments in favor of having an exercise routine.

If you're not already exercising, I hope the information in this chapter will persuade you to give it a try. Begin with a few minutes at a time. Don't try to compete with those slim young things on the television exercise broadcast or the commercials for exercise equipment. Be like Cindy, the woman whose exercise consisted at first of walking to the bathroom and back twice instead of once, doubling her daily exercise in the process.

• • • General Exercise Tips • • •

• Do small amounts of exercise at first. Doing anything, no matter how little, is better than doing nothing.

• Even if you can't walk or use a stationary bike, you can still exercise your arms. Start by using a small weight or a can of tomato paste. When that gets easy, use a bigger weight or a heavier can.

• Try to get your doctor to refer you to a physical therapist who understands fibromyalgia. Have the physical therapist watch how you move and help you avoid the mistake of "guarding" painful spots. Moving in a way that protects sore spots causes pain in other places because you use your muscles in unaccustomed and inappropriate ways.

• Ask the physical therapist to help you design an exercise routine that you can do on your own.

• Take a mild pain pill *before* you start to exercise to minimize postexercise pain.

• Increase your exercise time by thirty- or sixty-second increments when you feel up to it. If you overdo, you'll get discouraged and convince yourself you can't exercise.

• Have water handy and pause for a drink now and then while you're working out.

• Always stop before you get tired. You should feel you can still do a little more.

• Be aware that there are three aspects to a workout program: stretching, strengthening, and cardiovascular fitness.

• Find a videotape to guide you. (There are tapes for stretching, developing muscle tone, and increasing strength in the "Resources" section.)

• Aerobic exercise for cardiovascular fitness doesn't mean huffing and puffing. At its most vigorous, you should be able to carry on a conversation.

● ● ● ● ● ● ● ● ● ● ● ● ● ● ● ● ● ●

You don't need to work at the intensity of your "training heart rate" to benefit from exercise, but for those who want to try to achieve aerobic fitness, this is a goal worth pursuing to ward off heart disease and optimize energy. You can calculate your target heart rate by using the following formula: 220 minus your age in years minus your resting pulse. Multiply this figure by 0.6 and add your resting pulse. The resulting number is your goal in pulse beats per minute. To check your pulse, you can count beats for ten seconds and multiply by six. If you get to the point where you can reach this level easily and you want to go farther, you can change 0.6 to 0.7 or 0.8, but don't go higher than that.

Example: Say you are forty-five years old and your resting pulse is seventy-two beats per minute. Then:

$$220 - 45 = 175 - 72 = 103 \times .6$$
$$= 61.8 + 72 = 133.8 \div 6 = 22.3.$$

Therefore, your initial goal for aerobic fitness is twenty-two pulse beats in ten seconds. Remember, though, that it may take six months or even a year to reach this level. Be gentle and patient with yourself, as you would be with your best friend.

• • Stretch Before You Exercise • •

• Sit on the edge of a bed or on a chair and lean forward, letting your arms and, if possible, your head hang down. Don't push, just relax. Stay that way for a minute or two.

• Stand about one pace (thirty inches) away from a wall. Put your hands on the wall at shoulder height. With your feet flat on the floor, bend your elbows and let your straight body lean into the wall (like doing push-ups while standing). Repeat once or twice more.

• In the same position, put one foot ahead of the other, keep both feet flat on the floor, and lean into the wall again, once or twice. Switch feet and do it again.

• • • Guidelines for Walkers • • •

• Walking is wonderful exercise. It can be done outside or inside, or in a heated pool. Even when you can't leave your home, you can walk around a room or up and down the hall.

• If you're a beginning walker, walk for no more than five minutes the first time, and increase by no more than five minutes a day when you're ready to increase. Walk on level or gently sloping ground, not on hills.

• The speed at which you walk isn't important; it's the length of time that matters.

• If you live near a mall, call the management office and find out whether the mall opens early for people who want to walk. Many malls have organized walking clubs, and you'll have a flat, smooth surface on which to walk. Walking during shopping hours isn't the same; you have to slow down for browsers and can't work up a steady rhythm, which is important if you are to achieve maximum benefit.

• • • • • • • • • • • • • • • • •

For most people, the best time of day to exercise is late afternoon, four or five hours before bedtime. If you exercise later than that, you're apt to be overstimulated when it's time to turn out the lights. Aside from that precaution, any time of day is acceptable. Some choose to capitalize on the added burst of energy and mental clarity that follows exercise by making it the first thing they do in the morning.

There are two schools of thought on whether or not you should exercise every day. It is typical with FM to feel more aches two or three days after exertion than on the day you exercise. I find that if I skip a day, I'm more sore the next day than I would have been had I exercised each day. This is not true for everyone. Experiment and monitor yourself, then make your own decision. You can have weak muscles that are sore, or strong muscles that are sore. Which will you choose?

The Role of Posture in Musculoskeletal Pain

When we hurt, we tend to adjust the way we move and hold our bodies to relieve strain on the sore places. Instead of using our muscles the way they are designed to be used, this practice of "guarding" sore spots usually makes things worse. Over months or years, we may adjust our posture in ways that cause pain in places that might otherwise not hurt. Tension and the stress of living with chronic pain can have a similar effect. For example, when I look around a roomful of people with fibromyalgia, I usually find that most have their shoulders hunched up toward their ears. It's no coincidence that most people who have fibromyalgia experience shoulder and neck pain. Some of our pain is undoubtedly caused by the way we hold ourselves.

A friend told me about a form of bodywork known as the Alexander Technique and introduced me to someone who teaches it. Alexander teachers, as they are called, do not claim to be therapists, although they go through 3,000 hours of training to become certified. The technique was first developed by an actor who found himself losing his voice and discovered that his posture on stage was causing him to tighten his throat. Eventually he codified what he had taught himself in his effort to solve his problem (and save his career) and began teaching others his technique. Today Alexander teachers are popular with professional musicians and others whose work requires them to assume unnatural positions for long periods. Typists and computer operators are another prime population that can benefit from the Alexander Technique. There is an organization of certified Alexander teachers that can tell you whether there is one in your area (see "Resources").

Alexander lessons are so gentle that you may think nothing is happening, but your muscles and nerves will know differently. Usually, lessons are "taught" with the student lying on a massage table and the teacher making gentle adjustments to the student's body position. Some people benefit from verbal instruction as well; others don't. At the time of my first lesson, most of my pain was in my shoulders. I mentioned this to my Alexander teacher, and, in the course of the lesson, she gently moved my shoulders into their natural position. I felt the difference, lying down, immediately, but it became much more pronounced when I stood up. Throughout the week that followed, every time my shoulders started to hunch up again, I consciously moved them back to where they belong. My pain was greatly relieved almost immediately, although a good Alexander teacher will disclaim any ability to cure anyone.

I invite you to try the following exercise. (This is *not* an Alexander lesson. I'm not qualified for that. It is just a small example of what I have learned.) If your shoulders are not already in a defensive mode (raised and brought forward toward your chest), try to assume that position and see how it feels, physically and mentally. If they are already in that position, try moving them downward and toward your back and see how that feels, physically and mentally. If you can manage to get your shoulders into their natural position you will be wider across the shoulders, your chest will be more prominent, your elbows will point backward instead of out to the sides—and I think you will feel mentally clearer, more confident, and more alert. The way you feel mentally and emotionally affects your posture, but your posture also affects the way you feel.

If you can't assume this position without forcing it, please don't do it; you don't want to risk injuring yourself. If, however, you can do the exercise, you'll get some idea of what I experienced the first time my Alexander teacher put my shoulders where they belong. That was two years ago. I don't go for lessons anymore. Alexander lessons are not meant to go on forever, and you'll know when it's time to stop. I like the fact that Alexander lessons teach you something you can do for yourself for the rest of your life, rather than fix you up for a week, after which you need another session. I know of one woman who completed her work in six months and another who has been going for two years and still has a lot of work to do.

My shoulders no longer hurt, and I can raise my arms over

my head for the first time in years. I have learned to stand tall and in balance. I can stand at a party for two or more hours at a time without pain. If ever that stops being true, I'll know it's time to go back for a tune-up.

The Feldenkreis and Traeger methods have similar goals, and you may be able to find practitioners where Alexander teachers are not available. What's important is that these techniques teach you something of lasting value, and don't require you to hurt as you learn. All three of these techniques are taught both in one-on-one sessions and in groups. My advice is to start with individual sessions and make sure your instructor is familiar with fibromyalgia and how it affects you. You shouldn't have to try to keep up with a group of NDAs while you're working to improve your own physical well-being.

10

Standing Up for Yourself

You already know more than most people do about fibromyalgia—you're living with it and you know how real it is. Don't let anybody take that away from you. Listening to people who deny your reality can make you feel crazy. You don't have to convince anybody. Your time is more valuable than that, and you don't have energy to waste. You need all the time and energy you can muster in order to take charge of your own health care, your physical condition, and your mental well-being. This chapter is devoted to ways to stand up for yourself even though standing up at all may be a difficult thing for you to do. There are clearly defined steps to take, in whatever order makes the most sense to you. You don't have to complete all the steps before you start seeing beneficial results. Even the smallest step will bring you closer to your goal, a life that is rich and full, although it may be somewhat different from the one you knew before your diagnosis.

Learn Everything You Can

If you want basic FM information and confirmation that you are not alone in this, I suggest you start with my book *Fibromy-*

algia: A Comprehensive Approach—What You Can Do About Chronic Pain and Fatigue. It's the book I wanted to find when I got my diagnosis. I made it easy to read, especially for people who have cognitive problems. For nonmedical readers who want more technical detail, I recommend *The Fibromyalgia Help Book* by Jenny Fransen, R.N., and I. Jon Russell, M.D. Details on both books appear in the "Resources" section.

At least twenty-five other books on FM exist, some written for medical professionals, some for people who have the disorder, and some for those who care for them. There are books on fibromyalgia humor, for the well spouses of people who have fibromyalgia, and even a book of easy-to-prepare recipes. In the "Resources" section I explain how to use the Internet to find all of these books, and more. Also in that section you will find information on medical journals and newsletters. You would do well to subscribe to one or more of these.

Keep your eyes open for notices about regional or national fibromyalgia conferences and attend one if possible. These conferences attract people who, like you, are finding their way toward a better quality of life. You will make valuable contacts and hear lectures from people engaged in fibromyalgia research. Such conferences can be a bit overwhelming at first, but if you accept the idea that you may not be able to attend every session (few people do) and are not required to absorb every single bit of information (no one can), you will find the experience beneficial and uplifting.

As you learn, keep your mind open to new possibilities. Don't worry that you don't understand everything you hear or read. If nobody has ever told you how smart you are, please let me be the first. You are the World's Foremost Authority when it comes to the most important subject in the world—your own body. Maybe you aren't aware yet of the depth of your own knowledge, but from now on you will be more mindful of what's going on with your body. Before long, your wisdom will be apparent.

Your job while you're learning is not to find the cure for fibromyalgia; it's to discover what makes you feel better. Treat yourself gently as you learn. Refuse to be overwhelmed. Encourage yourself along the way, just as you would encourage anyone embarked on a serious self-education program. Here is another place in which self-talk can be very beneficial.

Build Your Support System

While each of us must find our own way in this strange place to which fate, genetics, or plain rotten luck has assigned us, none of us can do it alone. We need the support of some person, or more than one person, who cares about us and will listen when we need to talk. We need someone who understands that his or her job is not to "fix" us, but only to listen and accept our feelings, hopes, and doubts. People who can help us kick around ideas and evaluate our plans get extra credit, but not if they see this kind of discussion as an opportunity for knockdown, drag-out intellectual argument. The last thing we need is one more reason to be pumping adrenaline.

As hungry as you may be for support, it's enormously important to protect those around you from being overwhelmed by your need to talk about what's happening to you and what you're learning. Even the most compassionate and loving person can reach a point of boredom and fatigue if all he or she ever hears from you is about fibromyalgia. One of fibromyalgia's gifts to us is a heightened sensitivity to the needs and feelings of others. Use that sensitivity to determine when it's time to change the subject to something light and neutral, or just to be quiet. If having someone with whom you can discuss FM is new to you, you'll make a few mistakes before you get the hang of pacing your needs in this area, but you'll learn. Grace and a sense of humor will help carry you through the initial stages of learning.

The luckiest among us will get the support we need from a

life partner. Some of us, however, live alone. And, like Helen, who discovered she was better off discussing fibromyalgia with relative strangers when her husband Joe's patience wore out, some will find what they need in a fibromyalgia support group. Some support groups are very good, and some are dreadful, with groups at every possible point in between. Call your local hospital and ask if there is a support group in the area. If there's a group you can get to, give it a try. You may be more comfortable if you call the leader before the meeting to introduce yourself. Calling gives you a first impression of the group, because groups tend to be much like their leader in outlook and focus. This is natural; a group that is out of sync with its leader will either get a new leader or stop being a group. Assuming your talk with the leader doesn't discourage you completely, go to the next meeting.

Figuring out if the group is right for you is easy: Do you feel better after the meeting than you did before? Did you learn one useful thing, pick up one new idea, see one ray of hope? If the answer to any of these questions is yes, go back to the next meeting. If not, look for another group. And keep working to find an individual who will listen and understand.

Assemble Your Medical Team

Think of the people who will help you take charge of your FM as a committee, with you as its chair. Committee members will be your primary physician and any specialists and auxiliary medical personnel you and your physician agree should be involved. Your primary support person or someone you select as an advocate rounds out the team. If you don't already have a health care professional you can work with, finding one should be one of your highest priorities, especially if you have severe pain or are unable to get restorative sleep. You need someone who can write prescriptions, refer you to appropriate specialists when necessary, and whom you can consult about auxiliary services such as physical and occupational therapy and bodywork.

Your primary physician need not be a rheumatologist, although rheumatologists are most often thought of as the doctors who specialize in fibromyalgia. This is true mainly because rheumatology is the first specialty most people think of when they are dealing with musculoskeletal pain. A rheumatologist is less likely than a family doctor or internist to be able and willing to coordinate your care and to monitor your medications and progress—and these are the most important services a doctor can provide to you (next to getting you the sleep and pain relief you need in order to think clearly and chart your own plan for returning to health). One woman I know was taking thirteen different drugs, prescribed by four different doctors, none of whom knew of the others' existence. I learned of this when she told her support group that her liver was failing. Each of the four doctors was a specialist in a different field. None had ever asked her if she was taking any medications other than those he prescribed, and this poor woman didn't know she should offer that information.

If you don't now have a doctor who can serve as your primary physician, you may want to find one. Support groups are good for this purpose. You will usually encounter a few people who are satisfied with their doctors and who will provide their names. Word of mouth is the best way to locate a fibro-aware physician. If that doesn't work, get in touch with one of the organizations listed in the "Resources" section that maintain lists of doctors who at least know fibromyalgia exists. Or ask your local hospital or medical center to provide some names. If all else fails, you can turn to the yellow pages of your telephone book. When calling a doctor's office, be sure to ask the person who answers the phone if the doctor treats people with fibromyalgia. If the person says, "Fibro *what?*" say good-bye and hang up. If the receptionist never heard of it, the doctor doesn't treat it.

No one can guarantee that you'll hit it off with a particular doctor, but your chances will improve if you keep a few things in mind. First and most important, Western culture tends to elevate doctors to the level of gods. Don't fall into this trap. Even though some doctors accept this view of themselves, no single human being can know everything there is to know in a given field, not even the field of his or her specialty. If you've done your homework before your visit, you may know things about FM that the doctor doesn't know. It must be very difficult to sit across the desk from someone sleep-deprived and in pain and not have a ready answer to that person's problems. Talking about this, a dentist I know who gave up her own practice when arthritis crippled her hands (she also has fibromyalgia) said, "Believe me, even the best doctors get scared that they are missing something. My doctor friends know they are not gods; they are just bright people doing the best jobs they can. It doesn't make them happy that they can't cure fibromyalgia patients."

If you can approach the doctor in the spirit of "Let's see what we can figure out together to make me feel better"—implying that you don't expect the ultimate solution on the first try and are willing to be patient while you experiment with more than one approach—you'll help the doctor help you. Like the rest of us, doctors tend to behave in response to others' expectations. If you act as though you expect a quick fix, you'll almost surely get a prescription, but it may not be what you really need. If, on the other hand, you indicate that you're in this effort for the long haul, the doctor will be better able to proceed in an orderly way to try various solutions until the right one is found.

Second, while most doctors go into medicine genuinely hoping to help people, most soon learn that there is not enough time in the day to provide emotional support as well as medical treatment. Thus, they come to see their role as involving diagnosis and treatment. This may disappoint you. You're in pain and are naturally feeling vulnerable and needy. You want someone to listen to your sorrow and fear and offer comfort, but few doctors, even those who would like to provide that kind of support, can do so. If, instead, you approach the doctor as a source of information and advice—a consultant, in a sense—you're more likely to have a successful relationship. There are other, less expensive ways to get emotional counseling and support.

Few doctors know what it's like to live with a chronic condition. What may seem like indifference may simply be lack of knowledge of the implications of fibromyalgia. You can help both yourself and the doctor's other FM patients by offering insights into the problems you face daily, but do this in small increments. Perhaps bring up one problem per visit, ideally with a description of how you are attempting to handle it, always leaving room for the doctor's question or comment. Both of you may learn from the exchange.

Like most of us, doctors have certain prejudices. Some have been so thoroughly indoctrinated to accept only information that has been proven scientifically that they discount anything else. My favorite illustration was provided by a veterinarian a few years ago. Veterinarians receive the same kind of rigorous training that medical doctors receive, only they work on animals instead of human beings. When I took my old dog Mario for a booster shot, we were in the midst of a hot, damp summer and fleas were particularly rampant. I coaxed Mario onto the examining table. The vet looked him over and said, "This is the first dog I've seen this summer that isn't infested with fleas." I told the doctor, "We give him brewer's yeast. The fleas don't like the smell and they stay away." "Oh," said the vet with a dismissive wave of his hand, "that doesn't work."

This phenomenon accounts for the existence of so much doubt among doctors as to the existence of fibromyalgia, and the insistence of some that we are nothing but a bunch of hypochondriacs. Hypochondria is a psychological illness in which the patient complains of symptoms for which no physical explanation can be found. Typically the hypochondriac patient is anything but pleased when laboratory tests show no abnormalities. Do you remember when you'd never heard of fibromyalgia but knew you weren't well? You went to a doctor, passed all your tests with flying colors, and weren't happy to be told there was nothing wrong with you. That makes you a hypochondriac by definition, in the view of some doctors.

It may help you to know that fibromyalgia is far from the first ailment for which doctors blamed the patients until laboratory research identified a cause. Consider the following quotation on epilepsy from *Textbook of Medicine*, by Russell L. Cecil, A.B., M.D., Sc.D., a standard medical school text in the 1940s:

> Between attacks the frank epileptic is usually a constitutional psychopath of the most disagreeable sort . . . self-centered, unable to grasp the viewpoint of others, and childishly, uncomprehending when forced to accept the opposite view. . . . Institutional treatment properly directed along strictly modern lines affords the best possible means of handling [epileptics]. . . . In properly conducted institutions the epileptic . . . [is] taught to view his malady in its proper light.[21]

Writing about diabetes in the 1961 edition of the *Popular Medical Encyclopedia*, Morris Fishbein, M.D., said:

> A famous Viennese physician classified diabetics into two types—those who are blamable and those who are blameless. Most people who develop diabetes are fat before they get it. Dr. E. P. Joslin says that any ten diabetics put together weigh a ton before they develop the disease. He calls these fat people blamable diabetics because they would not have had diabetes if they had kept their weights down to normal. The blameless diabetics are the children who develop the disease, and most of those are under ten years of age.[22]

Fishbein was no backwoods physician without the advantages of exposure to modern medicine. For twenty-five years before he wrote the *Popular Medical Encyclopedia*, he edited the American Medical Association's magazine, *Hygeia, the Health*

Magazine, which was later renamed *Today's Health.* Fishbein also wrote in the *Encyclopedia:*

> Scientists also recognize what is called psychogenic pain, which is wholly mental. Such pain does not possess the qualities of pain that are associated with pain that is physical. The psychogenic pains are vague, they are irregular in their appearance, they are likely to be exaggerated in description, and they are usually accompanied by signs of excellent health otherwise. Pains that are more psychogenic than physical are likely to clear up when the mental reason for the pain disappears.[23]

These words were published in 1961, not in the Dark Ages. Many doctors practicing today were in medical school then, and many more have been trained by those who were trained at that time. Keeping this in mind the next time you hear of a doctor who "doesn't believe in fibromyalgia" may give you a different view of that doctor's competence.

It is unfortunate that many doctors think that everything that can be known about human health is already known. That is definitely not so. Until the mid-1990s, stomach ulcers were thought to be caused by stress. When an Australian doctor discovered *H. pylorus,* the bacterium that causes ulcers, medicine's view of the disease was altered. Yet there are still doctors practicing today who have never heard of this demonstrated fact, and patients who are told to see psychiatrists, to take medicines that coat their stomachs and deprive them of needed nutrients, and to stick to a bland diet rather than being prescribed the ten-day course of antibiotics that would cure them.

I sympathize with you if you're dissatisfied with your doctor but afraid to find a new one. Some positive self-talk can help in such a situation. You don't have to leave the doctor you have until you've found one more suitable, so seeing a new doctor won't leave you without medical care if the visit doesn't yield positive results. Seeking a doctor better able to help you is not an act of disloyalty to your current physician. Moreover, it is an important step on the way to improving the quality of your own life, which should be your most important consideration. There is a saying among people who earn their living in sales: Each "no" brings you one step closer to your next "yes." I suggest that each nonproductive meeting with a new doctor brings you that much closer to the right doctor for you. What's really at risk in meeting a new doctor is the price of the office visit. While that's not trivial, it fades in importance compared to your need and desire to be as healthy as you can be.

Take the time required to prepare for your meeting with a doctor you hope to hire for your medical care committee. Write a brief medical history listing in separate sections childhood illnesses and immunizations, major illnesses, surgeries, injuries, and allergies. Add a section for fibromyalgia symptoms, including date of onset of each, what you tried, and with what results. You probably have a great deal to say about each of these categories. Write it all out, but then edit carefully, omitting as many extraneous details as you can and leaving out descriptive words such as *severe, terrible,* and so forth. Be as factual and unemotional as you can. Although you're talking about yourself, your written information will make the best impression if you can present it in a detached manner, somewhat the way a doctor would write to another one about a patient, except that you'll use your own words, not medical jargon.

Then write a cover letter in which you introduce yourself as a human being, not a medical case. Again, be as concise as you can be, but let the doctor know of your distress at the situation in which you find yourself. Stress your desire to feel well and be able to function fully. Say that you have done what you could do to educate yourself about fibromyalgia, and that you are looking for someone who will help you learn more about self-management of the condition. Mention the actions you are taking to improve your well-being, and add that you are open to suggestions of more and better things to try. In doing this, you will make it clear that you are trying hard to take a positive approach and are not expecting a miracle on the first visit. If that doesn't show the doctor that you are a person worthy of help and capable of being helped, nothing will and you may as well stay with the doctor you are currently seeing.

If there's time, mail your letter and history to the doctor in advance of your appointment. Go to the appointment with a written list of two or three of your most pressing questions or problems. You'll probably have to fill out the doctor's own medical history questionnaire in the waiting room. Be sure that the material you prepared accompanies that form when the nurse gives it to the doctor. Try to meet the doctor while you are still fully clothed so that the first impression you create is of an adult in control of herself and trying to be well, not a sick, submissive person in a johnny. If you must disrobe first, at least be seated in a chair and not up on the examining table when the doctor walks in, stand up if you can, and offer to shake hands. This is the way you establish the relationship as one of adult to adult, rather than child to parent or, perish the thought, worshiper to a god.

Over several decades and more disappointments than I can count, I have learned to view my relationship with my doctor as a business relationship in which I am buying the doctor's time and advice based on her training and knowledge. I once asked my doctor—before I signed on to her service—if she would have a problem knowing that I intended to use her as my consultant and make my own decisions. She beamed. "That's exactly what I want, too," she said. When we meet to solve a health problem of mine, we know that we are bringing different perspectives and collections of knowledge to bear, and we work as a team, respectful of each other.

The third member of your basic medical team is your advocate. This should be someone you trust: your spouse, life partner, a family member, or a good friend. Most often your advocate will be an almost-silent partner, available if you need help and someone with whom to explore ideas and strategies. When you are in crisis, however, you may want your advocate to speak for you and will surely want her or him to accompany you on your visit to the doctor. My husband drove me to the visit during which I got my FM diagnosis because I was too sick to drive myself. I wanted him in the examining room with me because I was in such bad shape cognitively that I didn't trust myself to remember what the doctor said. Since then there have been times when I needed his company, but I make sure that he knows the results anytime I see or speak with my doctor. He has my medical power-of-attorney, a legal form on file in my medical records with a copy at home where he can find it. He has the authority to make decisions on my behalf if ever I am unable to speak for myself. I find it very reassuring to have this arrangement and recommend it to you.

Think of this triad—your doctor, your advocate, and you—as the steering committee that oversees your health care. If you think you need a referral to a specialist, that might well be a decision for the steering committee. The right doctor for you is one willing to recognize when he or she lacks the specific knowledge you need and to refer you to a specialist for a consultation. In the best of circumstances, though, the specialist will suggest a course of treatment or action to you and your physician but will not continue to treat you unless the situation demands it. It is of utmost importance that your primary physician know the details of your treatment. Otherwise, you risk having prescriptions that conflict with each other, possibly causing adverse interactions. There are exceptions to this requirement of extensive communication between primary physician and specialist, however, in the case of a referral for emotional counseling—often a very good idea if you are new to this diagnosis and need some time to express anger and grief. Also, auxiliary medical professionals such as physical and occupational therapists don't need to report in detail, but your primary doctor should know if you are seeing them.

The arrangement I have described, in which one doctor takes overall charge of your health care, is the model of the health maintenance organization (HMO), but you needn't belong to an HMO to make it work for you. HMOs have come in for a large portion of criticism in recent years, not all of it fair or accurately reported in the news media. It's true that there are some HMOs that operate as profit-making businesses, rewarding the doctors who treat the greatest number of patients in the shortest amount of time and order the fewest laboratory tests. But that is the exception, not the rule, and state and federal regulations are making that practice less and less common.

Whether you belong to an HMO or are a fee-for-service patient with a doctor in private practice, you need to stand up for yourself in all matters pertaining to your medical care. You have the right to receive respectful, considerate, nondiscriminatory treatment at all times, to take part in all decisions pertaining to your medical treatment, and to get a full explanation, in terms you can understand, of the pros and cons of any course of action. If you ask to be referred to a specialist and your primary doctor refuses, you have a right to know why. In an HMO you should have the right to appeal to a third party or doctor-patient committee set up for the purpose. It's important for you to know the procedures for making an appeal before a situation arises in which that might be necessary. Your HMO probably has a booklet for new patients explaining policies and procedures. You should read it—not once, but every few months. Each time you'll absorb more information and probably see things you overlooked or forgot since the last time you read it.

Savvy HMO members make it their business to get to know the organization's member services representative or ombudsperson before a problem arises. One way to do that is to look around the HMO for something you can compliment. Perhaps the telephone operators always answer pleasantly and get your calls through quickly. Maybe there's a particular receptionist who is extra nice to you or a nurse who always goes that extra mile to make you feel comfortable. When you find something you can praise, call member services and ask for your representative. Be sure to write down the name when he or she answers the phone. State your compliment. If it is about a single individual, mention that person's name. If you make this call, you will not be forgotten. People in such customer service jobs hear complaints day in and day out. The rare person who calls to say something nice is like a ray of sunlight on a bleak day.

Your call will accomplish three things: You'll have the name of someone you can call if you need help; you'll have identified yourself as one who is not a chronic complainer; and you'll have brightened someone else's day. Not bad for a single telephone call.

Try Various Approaches

To improve the quality of your life with fibromyalgia, you have at your disposal a wide variety of medical and nonmedical tools, some of which you can begin using today. In this section you will find a summary of available options, each of which has been found useful by some people with fibromyalgia, organized by symptom or problem. (See table 10-1.) Don't attach any significance to the order in which items appear. There is no intention to suggest that any symptom or problem is any more or less important or serious than any other, or that any approach will be any more or less effective for you. It may be that the average person who has FM finds medicines A and B, supplements C and D, and physical activities E and F most helpful, but you are not average and you cannot base predictions concerning your reactions and success on the experience of any other person. Without getting overly technical, I've tried to explain how various measures are likely to interact with your symptoms. Now it's up to you to use your own true knowledge of your body, your intelligence, and your instincts to decide where to begin. The only serious mistake you can make now is to decide to do nothing.

Here are a couple of hypothetical situations to illustrate how to use table 10-1:

• Greta has almost given up hope of ever feeling better, but she doesn't want to continue feeling the way she does. She decides her first step will be to work on changing her attitude and trying to get into a more positive frame of mind. She starts by writing down all the positive things she can think of to tell herself, decides to read a book on cognitive behavioral therapy, and perhaps begins to look for a therapist she can see. She also decides to try some mild exercise in hopes of getting her brain's endorphins working to lift her spirits and relieve some of her pain.

• Pat decides his main problem is sleep. Since he sleeps alone, there is no one to tell him whether he seems to have obstructive sleep apnea. He makes an appointment with his primary care physician to discuss the possibility of a sleep study or some medication to help him conquer his nightly expectation that he will be unable to sleep restfully. He also embarks on a sleep hygiene program, hoping to be able to train his body to know when it's time to sleep.

Table 10-1: Available Options for Dealing with Fibromyalgia

Problem or Symptom	Possible Action
Nonrestorative sleep	Find out whether you have obstructive sleep apnea, bruxism, or nocturnal myoclonus; if you do, seek medical attention.
	Improve sleep hygiene
	Improve sleeping environment
	See your doctor about taking sleeping pills
	Work on pain relief
	Try winding-down routines at bedtime
	Avoid caffeine, alcohol, refined sugars
	Try nutritional supplements
	Look into tryptophn, 5-HTP, melatonin

Table 10-1 (continued)

Problem or Symptom	Possible Action
Nonrestorative sleep	Look into herbal sleep aids Try lavender aromatherapy Try positive self-talk Exercise four to five hours before bedtime
Musculoskeletal pain	Try DLPA See your doctor about taking pain medication Work on getting restorative sleep Start a gentle repetitive exercise program Learn stretching exercises and then do them See a physical therapist about "guarding" when you move Take lessons in the Alexander Technique, Feldenkreis, or Traeger methods See a professional massage technician Learn not to stiffen in response to pain Learn about substance P and the heightened pain response to counteract fear Don't let yourself get cold Don't let pain get bad before taking pain-relief preparations
Depression, anger, anxiety	Look into cognitive behavioral therapy Practice self-talk Let yourself grieve Talk to a counselor Try tryptophan, 5-HTP See your doctor about taking mood-altering drugs for emergency relief Work to minimize unnecessary stress Avoid alcohol, caffeine, refined sugars Optimize your nutritional intake Use biofeedback Avoid overstimulating environments Practice left-brain/right-brain task shifting Arrange always to have something to look forward to Find out whether you have a yeast overgrowth and, if so, make the necessary dietary changes

Table 10-1 (continued)

Problem or Symptom	Possible Action
Cognitive dysfunction	Conserve mental energy; don't worry about forgetting
	Work on deep-breathing techniques
	Work on getting restorative sleep
	Write down everything
	Set priorities
	Use a multisensory approach to learning and remembering
	Take ginkgo biloba and other nutritional supplements
	Do mental exercises
	Evaluate your standards
	Find out whether you have a yeast overgrowth and, if so, make the necessary dietary changes
Fatigue	Work on improving your sleep
	Pace yourself, be realistic
	Try gentle exercise
	Alternate work periods and rest breaks
	Learn to delegate and negotiate tasks
	Optimize your nutritional intake
	Take nutritional supplements
	Analyze and streamline your activities
	See your doctor to check your thyroid, hemoglobin levels
	Find out whether you have a yeast overgrowth and, if so, make the necessary dietary changes
Irritable bowel syndrome, constipation, diarrhea, stomach upset	Increase fiber intake (regardless of the problem)
	Improve nutritional intake
	Avoid refined sugars, keep fats low
	Try digestive enzyme preparation
	Eat more frequent, smaller meals
	Work to minimize avoidable stress
	Avoid caffeine
	Find out whether you have food allergies, particularly to milk and wheat; eliminate such substances from your diet
	Find out whether you have a yeast overgrowth and, if so, make the necessary dietary changes

When you choose where you want to begin, consult the Resources section for references to more information. The Index will direct you to the appropriate pages when you want to refresh your memory about the effect each action is expected to have on the symptom or problem.

Raise Fibromyalgia Awareness in Your Community

Join the effort to educate your neighbors and elected representatives about fibromyalgia. There's a vast lack of knowledge out there. Most people still have never heard of our condition. Many who have are under the mistaken impression that it is a form of hypochondria or malingering. Some insurance companies, unwilling to pay on disability claims when people claim FM as the cause, are using public relations techniques to undermine the credibility of people who have fibromyalgia. By spreading the truth about fibromyalgia as you know it, you will help not only yourself but also your sisters and brothers in pain.

When you have the opportunity, talk to people about fibromyalgia and what it does to people who have it. Keep yourself out of the story as much as you can, beyond mentioning that you are one of the millions of people who live with FM every day. That way, you won't sound as if you're complaining and looking for sympathy. Those are two perfectly valid things to do, but not with people who aren't part of your closest circle of family and friends. Appearing to complain gives people an excuse not to take seriously what you say.

I once heard a lecture on organizational development during which the speaker said something like this: "There is someone in every group—you know the type—who complains about being ill all the time but is in perfectly good health." I bit my tongue until the coffee break, then approached her and said, "About that chronic complainer you mentioned, how do you know he or she doesn't have fibromyalgia?" "Fibro what?" she said—a response familiar to those of us who have public education on our personal agendas. I had my opening, and I took the opportunity to give her about sixty seconds' worth of information, ending with the fact that while I look healthy as a horse I have it myself. I did this as lightly and informatively as possible, just as I would speak with someone who offended me with a racist remark or an ethnic joke. She took it well and clearly heard what I said. I may have helped the next person with FM that she meets. I surely helped myself avoid a simmering anger and the resulting stress. You can do this, too, when the occasion presents itself.

You can also exercise your rights as a citizen and communicate with your state and federal legislators to make them aware of FM. The state of Wisconsin in 1997 had a Fibromyalgia Awareness Day. How nice it would be if we got all our states to do that. The U.S. National Institutes of Health funds research into causes and cures of a wide variety of ailments. Fibromyalgia is one of them. Table 10-2 shows how your taxes were used in 1997 to fund research in fibromyalgia compared to chronic fatigue syndrome and rheumatoid arthritis.

Table 10-2: **NIH Research Funding for Chronic Fatigue Syndrome, Rheumatoid Arthritis, and Fibromyalgia in 1997**

Condition	Prevalence in U.S.	Total Dollars Spent	Dollars Spent per Person Affected
Chronic Fatigue Syndrome	1,500,000	$13,600,000	$9.00
Rheumatoid Arthritis	2,100,000	20,080,000	9.50
Fibromyalgia	3,700,000	2,350,000	0.64

Source: *Fibromyalgia Times,* published by the Fibromyalgia Alliance of America, fall 1997.

Why is so much less money going to fibromyalgia research when it is more prevalent than both chronic fatigue syndrome and rheumatoid arthritis combined? The reason for this inequity is simple: Our government doesn't know enough about fibromyalgia to put it in its proper place in the queue for research funds. It's up to us to make our elected representatives understand fibromyalgia's effect on individuals, their families, coworkers, and the U.S. economy. The Fibromyalgia Alliance of America and the Fibromyalgia Network, listed in the "Resources section," can send you information to pass on to your legislators, and provide suggestions on what to say. The more people who have fibromyalgia do this, the sooner research will find the answers we need to finish the job of improving the quality of our lives.

RESOURCES

In this section you will find a wealth of resources to help you on your way to a better quality of life. There are books, audio- and videotapes, organizations devoted to fibromyalgia and related conditions, companies that sell adaptive devices and other products, sources that provide names of doctors who know about FM, and a collection of resources on the Internet, where a great deal of information is available. Aside from my book and audiotape, which appear with my name attached, I am not associated with any of the companies or products listed here.

Books

Except where noted, these books may be ordered through any bookstore.

Berger, Stuart M., M.D. *How to Be Your Own Nutritionist.* New York: Avon Books, 1987.
The author demystifies nutrition, providing excellent guidance on everything from basic meal planning to therapeutic nutrition.

Burns, David D., M.D. *Feeling Good: The New Mood Therapy.* New York: Signet, 1992.
Do-it-yourself cognitive behavioral therapy. Practical advice, written exercises, and encouragement.

Chaitow, Leon, D.O., N.D. *Amino Acids in Therapy.* Rochester, Vermont: Healing Arts Press, 1988. A condensed and more technical version of Chaitow's *Thorsons Guide to Amino Acids* addressed more directly to physicians.

Chaitow. *Thorsons Guide to Amino Acids: What They Are, What They Can Do, and How to Use Them.* London: Thorsons/HarperCollins, 1991.
If you are interested in amino acid supplements, this is the book to read.

Cooper, Jack R., Floyd E. Bloom, and Robert H. Roth. *The Biochemical Basis of Neuropharmacology.* 7th ed. New York: Oxford University Press, 1996.
A graduate-level textbook on the actions of neurochemicals, written clearly and with little technical jargon, so that nonchemists can glean some useful information from it.

Crook, William G., M.D. *The Yeast Connection Handbook.* Jackson, Tenn.: Professional Books, Inc., 1997.
The author wrote the first popular book on yeast overgrowth in 1985. Many doctors discounted his information (and some still do), probably because the book blamed practically every illness known to humankind on yeast. Later editions have moderated that view somewhat. This is the latest edition.

Erdmann, Robert, Ph.D. *The Amino Revolution: The Breakthrough Program That Will Change the Way You Feel.* New York: Simon & Schuster, 1987.
Instructions for developing your own amino acid therapy program.

Fransen, Jenny, R.N., and I. Jon Russell, M.D. *The Fibromyalgia Help Book.* St. Paul, Minn.: Smith House Press, 1996.
Good technical overview and help for specific problems. Written for non-medical readers. Extensive bibliography. May be ordered from the Fibromyalgia Alliance of America (see Organizations).

Goldenberg, Don L., M.D. *Chronic Illness and Uncertainty: A Personal and Professional Guide to Poorly Understood Syndromes.* 1996. Order from the Fibromyalgia Alliance of America (see Organizations) or from Dorset Press, P.O. Box 620026, Newton Lower Falls, MA 02162; 617-243-5005.
One of fibromyalgia's best-known physicians, the husband of a woman who has FM, writes about his own experiences with chronic pain as sufferer and supporter. Subjects covered include fibromyalgia, chronic fatigue syndrome, back pain, insomnia, irritable bowel syndrome, migraine and other headaches, and depression.

McKenzie, Robin. *Treat Your Own Back* and *Treat Your Own Neck.* Waikanae, New Zealand: Spinal Publications, 1988. Order from Orthopedic Physical Therapy Products, Orthopedic Physical Therapy Products (OPTP), Annapolis Lane, P.O. Box 41009, Minneapolis, MN 55441; 800-367-7393.

Mindell, Earl. *Earl Mindell's Vitamin Bible.* New York: Warner Books, 1991.

Thoroughly researched and clearly written by a registered pharmacist with a Ph.D. For people who want to tailor their own vitamin intake to their particular needs. Gives symptoms of deficiencies, benefits of individual vitamins, and nutritional means of treating various health problems. Touches on minerals, herbs, and folk remedies.

Mosby-Yearbook. *Mosby's GenRx.* Published annually. Order from Mosby-Yearbook, 11830 Westline Industrial Drive, P.O. Box 46908, St. Louis, MO 63146-9934; 800-426-4545.
A reference volume on drugs, their characteristics, interactions, recommended doses. Produced independently, rather than by pharmaceutical companies, this is better than *Physicians Desk Reference.* It includes results of postmarketing studies not found in the PDR, as well as cost of therapy. Also available for computers on CD-ROM and 3½-inch diskettes.

Pascarelli, Emil, M.D., and Deborah Quilter. *Repetitive Strain Injury: A Computer User's Guide.* New York: Wiley, 1994.
A seven-point program for preventing and treating repetitive strain injuries, including proper keyboard techniques.

Pellegrino, Mark, M.D. *The Fibromyalgia Supporter.* 1997. Order from Anadem Publishing, 3620 N. High St., Columbus, OH 43214; 614-262-2359 or 800-633-0055.
Pellegrino, a doctor of physical medicine who has FM himself, has written several short books on the subject, including a cookbook. This one is addressed to people who live with or care for a person with fibromyalgia.

Quilter, Deborah. *The Repetitive Strain Injury Recovery Book.* New York: Walker and Co., 1998. Contains some material on prevention of repetitive strain injury, but the emphasis is on living with the condition and self-help recovery.

Reiter, Russell J., Ph.D., and Jo Robinson. *Melatonin: Your Body's Natural Wonder Drug.* New York: Bantam Books, 1995.
Reiter leads the field in melatonin research. This book is written for lay readers. Of special interest to people with fibromyalgia is the section on melatonin and sleep.

Sahelian, Ray, M.D. *5-HTP: Nature's Serotonin Solution.* Garden City Park, N.Y.: Avery, 1998.
This book explains how to combine 5-HTP and other natural supplements, herbs, hormones, and medicines to effectively treat medical and

psychiatric conditions, including depression, insomnia, anxiety disorders, PMS, migraine headaches, and overeating.

Shankland, Wesley E. II, D.D.S., M.S. *TMJ: Its Many Faces. Diagnosis of TMJ and Related Disorders.* 1996. Order from Anadem Publishing, 3620 N. High St., Columbus, OH 43214; 614-262-2359 or 800-633-0055. Excellent information on the treatment of pain caused by the temporomandibular joint dysfunction.

Shernoff, William M. *How to Make Insurance Companies Pay Your Claims: And What to Do If They Don't.* Mamaroneck, N.Y.: Hastings House, 1990. Advice from an attorney for people with medical and disability claims problems, as well as other insurance issues. Best read before trouble starts, the book is full of practical tips on how to fight back and win.

Trowbridge, John Parks, M.D. *The Yeast Syndrome.* New York: Bantam Books, 1986.
Comprehensive information on yeast overgrowth, including a diet plan and recipes.

Wells, S. M. *A Delicate Balance: Living Successfully with Chronic Illness.* New York: Plenum Publishing Corp., 1998.

Williamson, Miryam Ehrlich. *Fibromyalgia: A Comprehensive Approach— What You Can Do About Chronic Pain and Fatigue.* New York: Walker, 1996.

Periodicals

Fibromyalgia Network, P.O. Box 31750, Tucson, AZ 85751-1750; 520-290-5508. Quarterly newsletter published by a company that pioneered in FM information. $19 per year.

The Fibromyalgia Times, P.O. Box 21990, Columbus, OH 43221-0990; 614-457-4222. Fax: 614-457-2729. Published quarterly by the nonprofit Fibromyalgia Alliance of America. $25 per year. Contributors include some of the FM community's foremost practitioners. Well worth the subscription price, which includes a year's membership in the alliance.

Health Points, published by To Your Health, a Natural Goods Company, 11809 Nightingale Circle, Fountain Hills, AZ 85268; 800-801-1406. A free newsletter full of authoritative information on vitamins, herbs, nutrition, aimed at people with FM, chronic fatigue, arthritis, and other chronic pain conditions.

Journal of Musculoskeletal Pain, published quarterly by Haworth Press, 10 Alice Street, Binghamton, NY 13904; 800-429-6784. $32.40 per year. A peer-reviewed medical journal covering fibromyalgia, chronic fatigue, and myofascial pain syndrome. Most articles can be readily understood by nonmedical readers.

Audio- and Videotapes

"Fibromyalgia: How You Can Help Yourself," audiotape of a lecture I gave at St. Vincent Hospital, Worcester, Mass., in 1997. It contains material covered in *Fibromyalgia: A Comprehensive Approach* as well as information that came to light after I finished writing that book. Order from Miryam Williamson, P.O. Box 307, Orange, MA 01364. $10.

"Fibromyalgia and You," produced by I. Jon Russell, M.D., Ph.D., foremost fibromyalgia researcher. This videotape features leading experts, including Robert Bennett, M.D.; Laurence Bradley, Ph.D.; Carol Burckhardt, Ph.D.; Sharon Clark, Ph.D.; and Muhammad Yunus, M.D. Order from Fibromyalgia Information Resources, P.O. Box 690402, San Antonio, TX 78269.

"Fibromyalgia Exercise Video: Stretching," prepared by Sharon Clark, Ph.D., an exercise physiologist, and her husband, Robert Bennett, M.D., one of the best-known fibromyalgia practitioners. An excellent way to get started if you're not already exercising. Order from Oregon Fibromyalgia Foundation, 1221 S.W. Yamhill, Suite 303, Portland, OR 97205. $20 per tape plus $5 shipping for first tape, $3.00 for each additional tape. Order can be faxed to 503-273-8778.

"Fibromyalgia Fitness: Improving Muscle Tone and Strength." The second videotape in the series by Drs. Clark and Bennett. Ordering information same as above.

"Living Life Fully: MENTORS™ Daily Mental Training for People with Fibromyalgia" offers practical tools to help you transform what you are learning into daily habits, so you can better manage your symptoms and get on with your life. Order from Fibromyalgia, Portland Health Institute, 1515 SW Fifth Avenue, Portland, OR 97201-5445. $40 (includes $4 for shipping and handling).

Organizations and Information Sources

American Chronic Pain Association, P.O. Box 850, Rocklin, CA 95677; 916-632-0922. Nonprofit organization with more than 800 chapters in the United States, Canada, Mexico, Ireland, Russia, Australia, and New Zealand. Group sessions led by people with chronic pain provide support and teach pain management techniques. Workbook available to aid people with chronic pain regain control of their lives. Quarterly newsletter, relaxation tapes, training for group leaders.

American Fibromyalgia Syndrome Association (AFSA), c/o Fibromyalgia Network, P.O. Box 31750, Tucson, AZ 85751-1750; the nonprofit branch of the company that publishes *Fibromyalgia Network,* this organization raises funds for fibromyalgia research.

Center for Cognitive Therapy, 3600 Market Street, Philadelphia, PA 19101; 215-898-4100. Founded by Aaron T. Beck, M.D., the originator of cognitive behavioral therapy. Provides names of trained cognitive therapists.

Fibromyalgia Alliance of America, P.O. Box 21990, Columbus, OH 43221-0990; 614-457-4222. Membership organization that publishes *The Fibromyalgia Times.* Annual dues ($25) include subscription to newsletter. An abundant source of information sent on request at no charge. Write for a list of support groups and physicians familiar with FM, furnishing your postal address including ZIP code.

International Academy of Compounding Pharmacies, 800-927-4227, ext. 30. Any compounding pharmacy can provide you with L-tryptophan or 5-HTP by prescription. To locate a compounding pharmacy near you, call this organization. Be prepared to leave your name, address, and phone number. You will be called back by a person with the information. Some compounding pharmacies and nonprescription sources of these substances are listed under Catalogs and Products, below.

Interstitial Cystitis Association, P.O. Box 1553, Madison Square Station, New York, NY 10159; 212-979-6057.

Job Accommodation Network (a service of the President's Committee on Employment of People with Disabilities), West Virginia University, 918 Chestnut Ridge Road, P.O. Box 6060, Morgantown, WV 26506-6080;

800-526-7234, 800-ADA-WORK, 304-293-7186, 800-526-2262 (from Canada).

National Digestive Diseases Information Clearinghouse, 2 Information Way, Bethesda, MD 20892-3570. Information on irritable bowel syndrome.

National Fibromyalgia Research Association (NFRA), P.O. Box 500, Salem, OR 97308. Raises funds for fibromyalgia research. Send self-addressed stamped envelope (SASE) for a packet of information.

National Headache Foundation, 428 West St. James Place, Chicago, IL 60614; 312-878-7715, 800-843-2256. Information on headache and migraine. Relaxation tapes.

National Institute of Arthritis and Musculoskeletal and Skin Diseases (NIAMS), P.O. Box AMS, 9000 Rockville Pike, Bethesda, MD 20892; 301-495-4484. Part of the National Institutes of Health, responsible for granting congressionally appropriated research funds to research on fibromyalgia and other disease under its jurisdiction.

National Sleep Foundation, 729 Fifteenth Street NW, fourth floor, Washington, D.C. 20005; 888-394-7533. Information on sleep disorders and certified sleep laboratories.

North American Society of Teachers of the Alexander Technique, 3010 Hennepin Avenue South, Suite 10, Minneapolis, MN 55408; 612-824-5066, 800-473-0620. E-mail: nastat@ix.netcom.com. Information on the Alexander Technique, directory of teachers.

Pharmaceutical Manufacturer's Association, 800-762-4636. Phone for the *Patient Assistance Directory*, a free booklet listing drug companies that have compassionate care programs and procedures for applying. These programs are designed to benefit people of limited income who do not have prescription insurance coverage. For those who qualify, drugs are provided free of charge. Your doctor's assistance will be necessary in completing the forms.

Sjogren's Syndrome Foundation, 333 N. Broadway, Jericho, NY 11753; 516-933-6365. Fax: 516-933-6368, 800-475-6473. World Wide Web: www.sjogrens.com. Information for people with Sjogren's syndrome.

Thyroid Foundation of America, Ruth Sleeper Hall—RSL 350, 40 Parkman Street, Boston, MA 02114-2698; 800-832-8321. World Wide Web: www.tfaweb.org/pub/tfa. Newsletter, physician referrals.

Trigeminal Neuralgia Association. P.O. Box 340, Barnegat Light, NJ 08006. Send SASE for information.

Catalogs and Products

Adaptability, 75 Mill Street, P.O. Box 515, Colchester, CT 06415-0515; 800-566-6678. Tools to help with housework, cooking, dressing, and bathing; exercise devices; mobility aids.

Brentham Enterprises, 800-490-7483. Body Rite posture support, a harness with adjustable weights in small of back to keep back erect.

Bruce, 411 Waverly Oaks Road, P.O. Box 9166, Waltham, MA 02254; 800-225-8446. Adaptive devices, medical supplies.

Comfort Corner, P.O. Box 649, Nashua, NH 03061; 800-735-4994. Clothing and shoes designed for comfort. Obusforme seats and backrests.

Dr. Leonard's Healthcare Catalog, 42 Mayfield Avenue, P.O. Box 7821, Edison, NJ 08818-7821; 800-785-0880. Mobility aids include a folding cane, cane attachment for icy surfaces, and rolling seat; herbal preparations; long-handled duster.

Enrichments, P.O. Box 5050, Bolingbrook, IL 60440-9973; 800-323-5547. Adaptive devices for home, kitchen, bath; mobility aids; easy dressing clothes; easy-cook meals. Excellent selection of clever devices.

Footprints, 1339 Massachusetts, Lawrence, KS 66044; 800-488-8316. Mostly Birkenstock shoes and sandals. This company allows you a six-month test period and accepts returns during that time for a full refund. A truly remarkable policy.

Intelli-Health Healthy Home, 960C Harvest Drive, Blue Bell, PA 19422; 800-394-3775. Devices for pain and stress relief; air purifiers and other items for people with allergies.

Janice Corporation, 198 U.S. Highway 46, Budd Lake, NJ 07828-3001; 800-526-4237. Items for people with allergies; bedding, bathroom articles, clothing, skin care, and grooming.

Lang Co., 714-530-3300. E-mail: glang@makura.com. Buckwheat pillows that have not been chemically treated.

L-tryptophan and 5-HTP Sources

Compounding pharmacies include:

College Pharmacy, 833 N. Tejon Street, Colorado Springs, CO 80903; 800-888-9358, 719-634-4861. Fax: 800-556-5893 or 719-634-4513.

Hopewell Pharmacy and Compounding Center, 1 West Broad Street, Hopewell, NJ 08525; 800-792-6670. Fax: 800-417-3864.

Medical Center Pharmacy, 3675 S. Rainbow Boulevard, #103, Las Vegas, NV 89103; 800-723-7455. Fax: 800-238-8239.

Pathway, Inc., Ron Keech, R.Ph., 5415 Cedar Lane, Bethesda, MD 20814; 301-530-1112, 800-869-9160.

Super Value Pharmacy, 720 N. Industrial, Euless, TX 76039; 817-283-5308 (OK to call collect). Fax: 817-283-2821. E-mail: supval@aol.com.

Nonprescription sources of 5-HTP include:

Masseys, 128 West River Street, Chippewa, Falls, WI 54729; 800-462-7739. Brand-name shoes for women in a remarkable range of sizes, sold with a wear-them-for-thirty-days return policy.

Maxi Aids, P.O. Box 3209, Farmingdale, NY 11735; 800-522-6294. E-mail: sales@maxiaids.com. Website: www.maxiaids.com. Products designed for people who are physically challenged, arthritic, visually impaired, blind, deaf, hard of hearing; educational toys and games.

Metabolic Response Modifiers, 800-948-6296.
Priority 1, 800-443-2039.
Vitamin Research Products, 800-877-2447.
Note: These three listings are from the *Health and Healing* newsletter by Julian Whitaker, M.D., 800-539-8219. Priority 1 sells only to readers of Dr. Whitaker's newsletter or people referred by their physicians.

JCPenney Special Needs Catalog, P.O. Box 2021, Milwaukee, WI 53201-2021; 800-222-6161. Easy-dressing clothes for women and men, mobility aids, adaptive devices.

Priorities, 70 Walnut Street, Wellesley, MA 02181-2175; 800-553-5398. Web site: www.priorities.com. Unusually informative catalog for people who have allergies.

Sammons Preston, P.O. Box 5071, Bolingbrook, IL 60440-5071; 800-323-5547. Enormous selection of adaptive aids, therapeutic devices, home accessories for people with physical difficulties. Designed mainly for rehabilitation professionals, but the company sells to individuals as well.

Serenity, 180 W. Twenty-fifth Street, Upland, CA 91786; 800-869-1684. Catalog of relaxation tapes.

Sun Precautions, 800-882-7860. Sunproof clothing catalog for photosensitive people and those with sun allergies.

Thera Cane Company, 4250 Norex Drive, Chaska, MN 55318-3047; 800-456-1289. Makers of the Thera Cane, a device for self-massage, particularly useful for releasing myofascial trigger points.

The Internet

You don't need to be a computer genius to use the Internet's rich resources. In most cases, you don't even need to own a computer. Most libraries in the United States have Internet access, and more libraries are coming online every day.

The Internet consists of three segments—electronic mail (E-mail), newsgroups, and the World Wide Web—each of which has something of value for people who have FM. Here are some listings to help you get started.

E-Mail

FIBROM-L is an electronic mailing list dedicated to sharing information about fibromyalgia and support for those who have it and the people who care about them. When you subscribe to a mailing list, you begin receiving E-mail messages written by other subscribers. If you reply to a message, your reply is automatically sent to every other subscriber. You can also initiate your own message and receive replies from other list members. Because public libraries generally don't allow people to subscribe to E-mail lists, you'll need your own computer to become a member.

A word of warning: On a typical day FIBROM-L receives 150 to 200 messages. If you feel responsible for reading every one, you may quickly become overwhelmed by the volume of information. One way to handle this is to read only those messages whose subjects interest you. A line at the top of each message tells you the subject, making it easy to delete those you don't find relevant. Another technique is to read the first sentence or two of each message, giving yourself permission to delete it without reading any farther if it doesn't catch your attention.

Accepted procedure on an Internet mailing list is to read messages for a few days without responding (this is called "lurking") and then send a message introducing yourself. Some members will write back welcoming you to the list. Aside from introductions and welcome messages, most people write when they want to add to the pool of available information, ask questions, or request advice and support when they are having trouble. It is considered poor form to send messages that say nothing more than "me, too." People are apt to disapprove (and may tell you so) if you write about subjects that are not germane to fibromyalgia.

To subscribe to FIBROM-L, send an E-mail to

listserv@mitvma.mit.edu

with the message

subscribe fibrom-l your name

For example, Jane Doe would write

subscribe fibrom-l jane doe

When you subscribe, you will receive a form letter telling you about the history and purpose of the list, subscription options that are available to you, and how to unsubscribe. You should save this message for future reference.

There is also a mailing list called FMS-CHAT on which any subject is permissible. The subscription address is the same as the preceding one. The message should say

subscribe fms-chat your name.

Other mailing lists of possible interest:

Subject/Format	Send E-Mail to:	With the Message
Americans with Disabilities Act/questions and answers	listserv@vmi.nodak.edu	subscribe ada-law your name

Subject/Format	Send E-Mail to:	With the Message
Chronic fatigue syndrome/discussion	listserv@list.nih.gov	subscribe cfs-L your name
Chronic pain/discussion	listserv@sjuvm.stjohns.edu	subscribe pain-L your name
Hand pain, repetitive strain injuries	listserv@ucsfvm.ucsf.edu	subscribe sorehand your name

Newsgroups

Internet newsgroups are much like mailing lists, except that you don't have to send a subscription message and the information sent to newsgroups doesn't come to you as E-mail. Your Internet service provider (ISP) chooses which newsgroups to provide from the 10,000 or more available on the Internet. You may have to ask the company that provides your Internet service for a specific newsgroup. The ISP can also help you find newsgroups and tell you how to obtain the messages. Once you have downloaded the messages, you can read them and reply, just as you can with a mailing list. The difference is that you have to remember to download newsgroup messages, whereas E-mail messages come to you without any action on your part once you have become a subscriber to the mailing list.

The fibromyalgia newsgroup is alt.med.fibromyalgia. Some libraries do not furnish newsgroups that begin with the letters *alt*, which stand for "alternative," because some of the alt newsgroups are dedicated to material inappropriate for children and offensive to some adults. You can assure your local librarian that alt.med.fibromyalgia never transmits graphic images and that it is a responsible discussion of fibromyalgia.

Some of the other newsgroups that you may find interesting:

Subject	Newsgroup Name
Americans with Disabilities Act (duplicates the ada-law mailing list)	bit-listserv.ada-law
Chronic fatigue syndrome (duplicates the cfs-l discussion list)	alt.med.cfs

Subject	Newsgroup Name
Irritable bowel syndrome	alt.support.ibs
Migraine	alt.support.headaches.migraine
Sleep disorders	alt.support.sleep-disorder
Tinnitus	alt.support.tinnitus

The World Wide Web

The World Wide Web is the segment of the Internet with graphics. While newsgroups and E-mail lists provide information solely in alphanumeric form, on the WWW you can find drawings, diagrams, and photographs as well as text. To get around on the WWW, you need a piece of software known as a Web browser and a computer mouse or other pointing device.

Each screen of information that appears on the Web is called a page. Pages contain words and, often, pictures. A group of Web pages created by an individual or organization is called a Web site. Some of the words on a Web page are underlined. When you put your pointer over an underlined word or phrase a little hand appears, and if you click on the word or phrase you are taken to a different Web page that contains related information. The underlined area is called a link. Pictures often serve as links, too. If a picture is a link, the same hand appears when you put your pointer on the picture. Each Web page has its own address. You can get to a page by typing its address in a space provided by the Web browser or by clicking on a link to that page.

For example, the address of the front page to my Web site is

http://www.shaysnet.com/~wmson/

If you type that into your browser's address space while your computer is connected to the Internet, you will go to my Web site. There is a link that will show you the contents of the entire site. You can click on anything that interests you, and the related page will appear. One page consists of links to other fibromyalgia sites. If you start from there and spend enough time, you can visit hundreds of Web pages about fibromyalgia.

On the WWW, as well as everywhere on the Internet, you must keep your critical faculties sharpened to filter out information that is erroneous or self-serving. The Internet—mailing lists, newsgroups, and the Web—is designed for the free flow of information. There is no overseer of accuracy on the Internet. Sometimes this can be detrimental, if you don't exercise your own good judgment and listen to your instincts. For example, before the diet pill fenfluramine was removed from the marketplace because of its ill effects on the heart and lungs of some who took it, that drug combined with phentermine (fen-phen) was promoted widely on the Internet through health-related mailing lists and newsgroups by a doctor who claimed he could use them to cure a host of diseases, including fibromyalgia, AIDS, and cancer. There was no law to prevent this kind of self-promotion, and this doctor actually recruited many patients on the Internet, took their money, and prescribed for them without ever seeing them in his office. There is also no law that prevents a person from putting the letters *M.D.* after his or her name and claiming to be a physician when that is not true. If you're going to take medical advice from an Internet doctor, be sure to check his or her credentials. Don't take anything on blind faith. The same is true of the fibromyalgia pages you come upon. If you look long enough, you may find a page that equates FM with Alzheimer's disease, which is both frightening and untrue.

However, as you explore the Web, you will learn to evaluate what you encounter. It would be a serious mistake to ignore its benefits simply because there are some rotten apples in the pile. You can find plenty of incorrect information in print or on the radio or television. Think of the Web as a visual talk show, and judge what you see accordingly.

You can also use the WWW to search for information. Web pages known as search engines allow you to type in a word or phrase of interest and see a list of Web pages on which relevant information appears. Another type of search engine helps you find Internet mailing lists and newsgroups that deal with your subject. To help you get started, here are four search engines.

Address of Search Engine	Comments
http://www.infoseek.com	Takes your search terms literally. If you type *fibromyalgia sleep dysfunction*, you will get a list of every page that contains any of these three words. Use the tips link for instructions. There is also a tutorial for new users.

Address of Search Engine	Comments
http://www.excite.com	Deals with concepts rather than specific words. If you type *chronic pain*, some of the pages on the list you get back will be about fibromyalgia, some about other chronic pain disorders.
http://www.dejanews.com	A search engine for newsgroups. Type in *fibromyalgia*, and you'll get some of the more recent messages sent to alt.med.fibromyalgia. You will also see messages about fibromyalgia that were posted on other newsgroups. You can click on the link to any of these messages to read them. You can also send E-mail to the author of a message that you see.
http://www.liszt.com	The Internet is full of puns, and the name of this page is one. It is a source of information on mailing lists (get it?). Type *fibro*, and you'll get information on FIBROM-L, FMS-CHAT, and the cystic fibrosis mailing list. Type *fibromyalgia*, and only FIBROM-L and FMS-CHAT will appear.

There are several million individual pages on the World Wide Web. Here are some that you will find most useful, in addition to my Web site.

Address of Web Site	Comments
http://www.shaysnet/com/ ~wmson	Information about *Fibromyalgia: A Comprehensive Approach*, this book, and articles on various FM topics including hypoglycemia, 5-HTP,

Address of Web Site	Comments
	and L-tryptophan, FM in children, yeast, and more. Links to other FM sites. You can order my audiotape from here.
http://www.myalgia.com	Site of the Oregon Fibromyalgia Foundation, headed by Robert Bennett, M.D. A generous helping of advice and information, medical articles, and an exhaustive bibliography of articles in medical journals. You can order Dr. Sharon Clark's exercise videos from here.
http://www. ncbi.nlm.nih.gov/PubMed/	PubMed is the National Library of Medicine's site for searching Medline, a database of journal article abstracts. A real treasure.
http://www. alexandertechnique.com	Information on the Alexander Technique.
http://www.FIBROM-L.org	Developed by some of the participants in the FIBROM-L mailing list.
http://www.csusm.edu/ public/guests/nancym/ fibromt.htm	Authoritative information on guafenesin as a treatment for FM.
http://www. sleepfoundation.org/	National Sleep Foundation site. Click on *sleep disorders*. There is no mention of FM, but the information is good.
http://www.rip-intl.com/as/ html/library.html	An encyclopedia of pain relief techniques, articles on pain control. Nothing specifically on FM here.
http://www.wco.com/ ~dietman/amino_rd.html	Information on amino acids.

Address of Web Site	Comments
http://www.rxlist.com	Information on prescription medicines.
http://www.usdoj.gov/crt/ada/adahom1.htm	Definitive information about the Americans with Disabilities Act.
http://janweb.icdi.wvu.edu/	Job Accommodation Network
http://www.tifaq.com	Information on typing injuries and links to related sites.

The above information was checked for accuracy in April 1998. Because the Internet is constantly changing, some addresses may have changed by the time you read this book.

Internet mailing lists and newsgroups don't care whether you use capital letters or lowercase ones, but the WWW is very fussy. If you are having trouble finding a Web site, make sure you have the upper- and lowercase letters exactly as they are given.

A complete list of Internet fibromyalgia resources could fill a book by itself. Many useful addresses have therefore been omitted. If you discover a Web site or other resource that you think should be included in a future edition of this book, please let me know. My E-mail address is <mwilliamson@reporters.net.>

NOTES

1. Russell, I. J. et al.: Elevated cerebrospinal fluid levels of substance P in patients with fibromyalgia syndrome. *Arthritis and Rheumatism* 1994; 37(11): 1593–1601.

2. Burckhardt, Carol S. et al.: Fibromyalgia and quality of life: A comparative analysis. *Journal of Rheumatology*, 20:475–479, 1993.
————: Quality of Life of Swedish Women with Fibromyalgia Syndrome, Rheumatoid Arthritis or Systemic Lupus Erythematosus. *Journal of Musculoskeletal Pain*, 1:3/4, 1993, 199–207.

3. These exercises are based on "Stretching Exercises for VDT Users," produced by the Communication Workers of America, AFL-CIO, District 1 with partial funding from the New York State Department of Labor.

4. Reiter, Russel J. and J. Robinson: *Melatonin.* New York: Bantam, 1995.

5. May, K. P. et al.: Sleep apnea in male patients with the fibromyalgia syndrome. *American Journal of Medicine* 1993; 94:505.

6. Hudson, J. I., et al.: Fibromyalgia and Eosinophilia-Myalgia Syndrome. *Journal of Musculoskeletal Pain* 1995; 3(1).

7. Manders, D. W., Ph.D.: The FDA ban of L-tryptophan: Politics, profits, and prozac. *Social Policy*, winter 1995; 26(2).

8. I recommend the following articles: Spinweber, C. L.: L-tryptophan administered to chronic sleep-onset insomniacs: Late appearing reduction of sleep latency. *Psychopharmacology* (Berl) 1986; 90(2):1515. Hartmann, E.; J. G. Lindsley; C. Spinweber. Chronic insomnia: Effects of tryptophan, flurazepam, secobarbital, and placebo. *Psychopharmacology* (Berl) 1983;80(2):13842. Demisch, K.; Bauer, J.; Georgi, K.: Treatment of

severe chronic insomnia with L-tryptophan and varying sleeping times. Department of Psychiatry, Hospital of the University of Frankfurt. *Pharmacopsychiatry* 1987 Nov;20(6):2458. Hartmann, E.: Effects of L-tryptophan on sleepiness and on sleep. Review Article: 14 Refs. *Journal of Psychiatric Research* 1982–83;17(2):10713.

9. For a complete description of this study, see the May 1996 issue of the journal *Lancet*.

10. Nielson, W. R.; C. Walker; G. A. McCain: Cognitive behavioral treatment of fibromyalgia syndrome: Preliminary findings. *Journal of Rheumatology* 1992;19:98–103.

11. Sprott, H.; H. Kluge; S. Franke; G. Hein: Altered serotonin levels in patients with fibromyalgia. *Journal of Musculoskeletal Pain* 1995;3:65.

12. McDermid, A. J.; G. B. Rollman; G. A. McCain: Generalized hypervigilance in fibromyalgia: Evidence of perceptual amplification. *Pain* 1996 Aug;66(2–3):133–44.

13. Dunbar, R.: *Grooming, Gossip, and the Evolution of Language*. London: Farber and Farber, 1996.

14. Berger, S. M., M.D.: *How to Be Your Own Nutritionist*. New York: Avon, 1993.

15. Bland, J., ed.: *Medical Applications of Clinical Nutrition*. Keats, 1983.

16. Chaitow, L.: *Amino Acids in Therapy*. Rochester, Vermont: Healing Arts Press, 1988.

17. Cowley, G. and A. Underwood: Surgeon, drop that scalpel. *Newsweek Extra*, winter 1997–98, p. 77.

18. Editorial. *Otolaryngology—Head and Neck Surgery* 1994 July; 111(1):1.

19. Trowbridge, J. P., M.D. and M. Walker, D.P.M.: *The Yeast Syndrome*. New York: Bantam Books, 1986.

20. Dunbar, R.: *Grooming, Gossip, and the Evolution of Language*. London: Faber and Faber, 1996, pp. 36–37.

21. Quoted in Szasz, T.: *Cruel Compassion: Psychiatric Control of Society's Unwanted*. New York: John Wiley, 1994, p. 58.

22. *The Popular Medical Encyclopedia*. New York: Doubleday, 1961, p. 172.

23. Ibid, p. 346.

INDEX

Accommodations (on the job), 33–40, 47
 scenarios, 38–39
Acetaminophen, 46–47
Acetylcholine, 6
Achilles tendon, 70
Acidophilus, 142
Activities, analyzing, 126
Acupuncture, 47
Adrenal glands, 5, 114, 130, 131
Adrenal system(s), 112
Adrenaline (epinephrine), 88, 130, 139, 143
 and hypervigilance, 117
 reliance on, to fight fatigue, 114–16
Adrenaline surges, 112, 115–16
Advocate, 167–68
Aerobic exercise, xii, 5, 147–48, 149, 151
Aerobic fitness, 151, 152
Air bag(s), 62
Airports/airplanes, 56–59
 early boarding, 57–58
Alanine, 137
Alcohol, 31, 46, 47, 58, 60, 77, 84, 88, 130, 137
Alexander Technique, 154–56
Alexander Technique teachers, 22, 68, 154, 155, 156

Allergens, 22
Allergies, 78, 79, 81
Alpha brain waves, 74
 intrusion into delta sleep, 75
Ambien, 79
Americans with Disabilities Act (ADA), 33–34, 37–40
Amino acids, 4, 136–40, 143
Amitriptyline (Elavil), 85
Analgesic drugs, 46–47
Anger, xii, 92, 100, 112, 113
Antibiotics, 141
Anticonvulsive drugs, 76
Antidepressants, 111
Antioxidants, 132
Antisnoring aid(s), 78
Anxiety, 92, 111, 112, 113, 114
Anxiety attacks, 114
Anxiety-related issues, 36
Arginine, 137, 140
Arms, 45
Arthritis, 8, 63, 110, 111, 175–76
Arthritis and Rheumatism (journal), 5
Artificial sweeteners, 130
Asparagine, 137
Aspartame, 59
Aspartic acid, 137
Aspirin, 46, 47
Assertive behavior, 100–101

Attendance issues (work), 35
Attitude, changing, 171
Autoimmune diseases, 74, 81, 135

B-complex vitamins, 131
   deficiency in, 47
Back muscles, relaxing, 27
Back pain
   at work, 40
Backs, 45
Bartholomew, Mel
   Square Foot Gardening, 25
Beck, Aaron T., 110
Bed
   moving in/getting out of, 89–90
Bed-making, 15–16
Benadryl, 79
Bending, 22
Beta-carotene, 132
Biochemicals, levels of, 3–4
Biofeedback, 116
Blood flow, 43
Blood sugar
   sudden drop in, 88
Blood sugar levels, 58–59, 89, 115,
   130, 131, 143
Body
   and mind, 106–26
   paying attention to, 15
Body chemistry, 6
Bodywork, 161
Bowel and bladder control issues,
   37
Brain, 126
   hemisphere theory of, 117–18
Brain chemicals
   and emotion, 113–14
Brain chemistry, 116
"Brain fog," 120–21
Bruxism, 76

Burns, David D.
   Feeling Good, 110

Caffeine, 130, 137
Calcium, 135–36
Cancer, 74
   immune system, 81
Candida albicans, 140–41
Cane(s), 57–58, 68–69
Caprylic acid, 142
Car travel, 61–65, 66
Carbohydrates, 4, 129–30, 142
Cardiovascular fitness, 151
Carnitine, 137
Carpal tunnel syndrome (CTS),
   43, 45
   splints for, 46
Cecil, Russell L.
   Textbook of Medicine, 164
Center for Cognitive Therapy,
   110
Cervical collar, 65
Chair(s), work, 40–41, 51
Chamomile, 81
Chemical imbalances
   and FM symptoms, 4–6
Chemotherapy, 74–75, 135, 143
Childhood, traumatic, 116–17
Children
   and cleaning, 12
   and food preparation, 16–17, 18
   and laundry, 22
   water bottles for, 20
Chiropractic physician, 47
Chronic fatigue syndrome, 110,
   175–76
Chronic headache-related issues,
   36
Chronic illness, 3, 6
   and relationships, 91, 92–93, 95,
   98

Chronic obstructive pulmonary disease, 8
Chronic pain, 6, 138, 154
Clauw, Daniel, 110
Cleaning, 11–16
Cleaning service, commercial, 14
Cleaning tips, 15–16
Cleanup, after-meal, 16–20
Clutter, eliminating, 12
Cod liver oil, 134
Coffee, 58
Cognitive behavioral therapy (CBT), 110–12, 116
Cognitive dysfunction
  sleep problems and, 74–75
Cognitive problems, 9, 119–24, 158
  coping with, 121–24
  cytokines in, 6
  sleep and, 73
Communication
  in relationship(s), 98–105
Complex carbohydrates, 129
Compost pile, 26
Compounding pharmacies, 80, 81, 138
Computer(s), 45, 46, 47–50
Computer work
  checklist for, 48–50
  tips for making more comfortable, 50–52
Concentration-related issues (work), 36–37
Conferences (FM), 158
Control of thoughts and feelings, 111, 112, 114
Cooking, 16–20
Corticosteroids, 141
Cortisol, 5
  abnormal release pattern, 76
CPAP (continuous positive airway pressure) machine, 75–76

Crutches, forearm, 69
Cubital tunnel syndrome, 43
Cumulative trauma, 45
Cumulative trauma disorder (CTD), 42
Cumulative trauma injury, 54
Cysteine, 137
Cystine, 137
Cytokines, 5–6, 74–75

D-L-phenylalanine (DLPA), 139–40
Dairy products, 4
Deep breathing, 121
Deep-tissue massage, 46
Defensiveness, 94
Defrosting, 15
Dehydration, 27, 58, 60
Delta sleep, 74, 79
  alpha-wave intrusion into, 75
Depression, xii, 81, 92, 106, 113, 136, 138
  cognitive behavioral therapy in treatment of, 110, 111–12
  exercise to combat, 145–56
  tips for lifting, 118–19
Depression-related issues, 36
Diabetes, 8, 135, 142, 164
Diagnosis, xi
Dialogue
  couples, 98–101
Diet, 114, 129–30, 142, 143
  balanced, 128
  and RSI, 47
Dietary needs
  and travel, 58–59, 67
Difficulty getting to sleep, 74
Digestive upsets, 73
Diphenhydramine (Benadryl), 79
Disability
  categories of, for disabled parking, 64

defined, 34
"qualified individual" with, 33
Disabled parking, 63–64
Discussing problems, 77
Disorientation while driving, 62
Division of labor, 91
Divorce, 91
Doctor(s), xiii, 160–69
  choosing, with RSI, 44–45
  dealing with, 9
  and disabled parking placard,
    63, 64
  finding, 161
  ignorance about nutrition, 127–
    28, 129
  information for employer(s) for
    job accommodations, 34–35,
    39
  relationship with, 167
  treatment of RSI, 46
Dopamine, 139
Driving, 61–65
Drugs, 137
  analgesic, 46–47
  mood-altering, 95, 114, 121
  opiate, 149
  prescription, 87, 143
  psychoactive, 144
  see also Medications
Dusters, 15

Earplugs, 66, 67, 77, 82
Efficiency, 6–8
Elavil, 85
Electroencephalographic (EEG)
  machines, 73, 75
Emotion(s)
  brain chemicals and, 113–14
  controlling, 109
  negative, 113
  see also Feelings

Emotional strains
  in relationships, 91–95
Employers, 34, 37–39, 40, 47–48
Endorphins, 140, 149–50, 171
Energy, lack of, 136
Energy conservation, 17, 124–26
Energy expenditure
  techniques regarding, 3
Entertaining, 27–29
Environment, sensitivity to, 117
Eosinophilia myalgia syndrome
  (EMS), 80
Epicondylitis ("tennis elbow"),
  42–43
Epilepsy, 164
Epinephrine
  see Adrenaline (epinephrine)
Erection, 96
Ergonomics, 6–7
Essential amino acids, 136–37
Essential fatty acids, 143
Euthymia, 87
Exercise, 137, 144
  benefits of, 147–53
  to combat depression and pain,
    145–56
  frequency of, 153
  in gardening, 25
  and RSI, 45
  while traveling, 58
  during work break(s), 52–54
Exercise program, 65
Exercise tips, 150–51
Exhaustion, 115
Eyeshades, 57, 66, 67, 82

Fainting, 130
Falls
  from fatigue, 57, 68
Family
  staying with, 67

Fatigue, xi, xii, 58, 130
  falls from, 57, 68
Fatigue-related issues (work),
  35–36
Fats (dietary), 129, 130, 131–32
Fatty foods, 77
Fear, 92, 93
  of pain, 107–8, 109
Feeling Good (Burns), 110
Feelings
  expressing, 92, 93, 99
  hidden, 100
  see also Emotion(s)
Feldenkreis method, 156
Fibromyalgia
  incidence of, xi
  mind and body in, 106
  options for dealing with,
    170–74
  and quality of life, 1–9
  and RSI, 45
  travel with, 55–72
  see also Symptoms (FM); Treat-
    ment (FM)
*Fibromyalgia: A Comprehensive Ap-
  proach* (Williamson), 1–2,
  157–58
Fibromyalgia Alliance of America,
  176
Fibromyalgia awareness, 174–76
Fibromyalgia Help Book, The
  (Fransen and Russell), 158
Fibromyalgia Network, 176
Fibromyalgia syndrome, xi-xii
"Fight or flight" response,
  114–15
Fishbein, Morris
  Popular Medical Encyclopedia,
    164–65
5-HIAA, 113
5-hydroxytryptophan (5-HTP),
  79, 81, 87, 138, 139, 149

FM
  see Fibromyalgia
Food, 125
  airline, 58–59
  amino acids from, 137
  in avoiding jet lag, 60
  deficient in nutrients, 128
  for entertaining, 28, 29
  inefficient body use of, 124,
    128, 142
  mineral content of, 135
  shopping for, 20–21
  source of serotonin, 4
Food preparation, 16, 18–19
  with houseguests, 30
Footprints (co.), 72
Footstool(s), 17
Fransen, Jenny, and I. Jon Russell
  Fibromyalgia Help Book, The, 158
Friends, 8, 28
  and cleaning, 14
  staying with, 67
Frustration, 92

Gardening, 24–27
Gardening tips, 26–27
Garlic, 142
Gift giving, 31
Ginkgo biloba, 121
Glucose, 130
Glucose tolerance, 140
Glutamic acid, 137
Glutamine, 137
Glycine, 137
Grief, 92, 95
  for losses, 93–94
Growth hormone, 140, 150
Growth hormone deficiency, 43,
  74
"Guarding" sore spots, 43, 150–
  51, 154
Guilt, 92, 93

Hand surgeon(s), 44
Hands, 44, 45
    numb, stiff, 19
Headache, 57, 58, 130
Health care organizations, dealing
    with, 9
Health maintenance organizations
    (HMOs), 168–70
Health status, 137
Help, asking for, 12
Herb teas, 81–82
Herbs
    as sleep aid, 81–82
Herpes virus, 140
Hip pain, 69
Histidine, 137
HIV/AIDS, 143
Holiday blues, 32
Holidays, 29–32
Home, 8
Home modifications, 23
Homeostasis, 117, 137
Honesty, mutual, 99–100
Hotels, 65–67
Houseguests, 29–30
Household activities
    taking pain out of, 10–23
Household cleanliness, 3, 11–23
Human growth hormone (hGH),
    5
    see also Growth hormone
Humidifier/vaporizer, 78
Hydroxyproline, 137
Hypochondria, 67, 163–64, 174
Hypothalamus, 149

Ibuprofen, 46
Immune system, 141
    compromised, 143
    sleep and, 74–75
Immune system hormones, 6

Inactivity, 43
Independence, 104
Insomnia, 74, 86, 136
    L-tryptophan in treating, 80–81
    subnormal tryptophan and, 138
Insulin, 130
Insulin-dependent diabetes, 8
Insurance companies, 174
Intercourse, 95, 96
Internal clock, 60, 61
Internal Revenue Service Form
    8826, 34
Internet, 2, 138, 158
Internet discussion group, 115
Isolation, 92, 93
Isoleucine, 137

Jet lag, 59–61
Job Accommodation Network
    (JAN), 35–37, 38
Job description, 33–34
Journal of Musculoskeletal Pain, 80

Kava kava, 81
Kitchen setup, 17
Kneeling bench, 27
Kynurenine, 138

L-tryptophan, 79–81
Laundry, 13, 21–22
Laundry detergents, perfumed,
    22
Lavender, 82, 85
Learn(ing) about fibromyalgia,
    xiii, 3, 157–59
Learning, multisensory approach
    to, 123
Leftovers, 18
Leucine, 137
Leukemia, 81
Lifestyle changes, xiii, 3

Lifting, 16, 34, 35, 41
Loss, sense of, 11
Losses, grieving, 93–94
Luggage, 56, 57
Lumbar support, 51–52, 58
    while driving, 62
Lupus, 8, 74
Luvox, 139
Lycine, 137
Lymphoma, 81
Lysine, 140

Magnesium, 135, 136
Mail-order catalogs, 31
Malaise, 115
Malnutrition, 128
Managing fibromyalgia, 2–3
MAO inhibitors, 139
Marplan, 139
Massey's (co.), 72
Mattress(es), 82
Medical history, 166, 167
    cover letter with, 166–67
Medical power-of-attorney, 168
Medical team, assembling,
    160–70
Medications, xii
    monitoring, 161
    promoting sleep, 78–81, 87
Melatonin, 60–61, 66
    as sleep aid, 81, 87–88
Memory, poor, 74
Memory loss, 119–20
Memory tasks, 124
Men
    life roles, 92
    obstructive sleep apnea in, 75
Mending, 22
Mental "background noise," 122
Mental confusion, 58, 115, 121

Mental energy
    conserving, 126
Mental life, 9
Mental responses to pain, 107–9
Metabolism, 4, 124, 128
Methionine, 137
Microscopic muscle tears, 5, 43
Mind
    and body, 106–26
    exercise for, 124
    and physical well-being, 9
Mineral supplements, 131,
    135–36
Modifications, 3
    of activities, 6–8, 45
    of home, 23
Moldofsky, Harvey, 73
Mood
    controlling, 107
    determined by thoughts, per-
        ceptions, attitudes, beliefs,
        111
    exercise and, 148, 150
    serotonin and, 138
    and stress, 110–19
Mood-altering drugs, 95, 114, 121
Mulch, 26
Multiple sclerosis, 74, 111, 135
Muscle-loosening techniques,
    85–86, 89, 109
Muscle pain, 73
Muscle pain and stiffness-related
    issues (work), 36
Muscle spasms, 43, 58, 136
Musculoskeletal pain, 161
    posture in, 154–56
Music, 15, 28, 84, 123

Naproxen, 46
Nardil, 139
National Research Council, 127

NDAs (people Not Diagnosed with Anything), 6, 59, 108–9, 121, 143, 156
Neck, 45, 65
Neck roll, 83
Needs, meeting each other's, 101–5
Negativity, 112
Neurochemicals, 136
Neurologist(s), 44, 75
Niacinamide, 132
Nightmare/night terror, 88, 130
Nocturnal myoclonus, 76, 87, 88
Nonsteroidal anti-inflammatory drugs (NSAIDs), 46, 47
Norepinephrine, 139
Nutrients
　absorption of, 142
　lost, 128
　responsibilities and risks, 143–44
Nutrition, 1, 8, 30, 114, 127–44
　basic principles of, 129
　and RSI, 47
Nutritional therapies, 143–44

Obesity, 74
Obstructive sleep apnea (OSA), 75–76, 78, 88, 171
Occupational hazards, 40
Occupational medicine doctor(s), 44
Occupational therapy/therapist, 161, 168
Oil-soluble vitamins, 131–32
Oral contraceptives, 141
Oral nystatin, 141
Organization, 123
Orgasm, 95, 96, 97
Orthopedist(s), 44, 70
Osteoarthritis, 8

Osteopathic physician, 47
Osteoporosis, 135
Overstimulation, 117
Oxygen deprivation, 43
　brain, 121

Pacing oneself, 16
Pain, xi, xii, 24, 106
　carriage and, 68
　exercise to combat, 52, 145–56
　and gardening, 26
　mental responses to, 107–9
　minimizing, 17
　response, to, 5
　in RSI, 43, 44
　and sexual drive, 95, 96, 97
　taking out of household activities, 10–23
　and walking, 68, 69
　work-related injury, 54
Pain perception, 113
　serotonin in, 138
Pain relief
　from cognitive behavioral therapy, 110
Pain sensitivity, 5, 40, 117
Painful places, "guarding," 43, 150–51, 154
Painkillers, 121, 144
Pancreas, 131
Panic attacks, 114, 130
Parnate, 139
Parties, 31, 32
Passionflower, 81
Peale, Norman Vincent
　Power of Positive Thinking, The, 106–7
Periodic limb movements of sleep (PLMS), 76
Phenylalanine, 137, 139–40
Phenylketonuria, 139

Physiatrist(s), 44
Physical condition, 43
Physical therapist, 69, 70, 150–51, 168
Physical therapy, 161
  and RSI, 45, 46
Pillows, 66, 82–83
Pineal gland, 81
Pituitary gland, 5, 74, 140
Pleasure
  maximizing moments of, 24–32
  sexual, 95
Podiatrist, 70
Popular Medical Encyclopedia (Fishbein), 164–65
Posture, 54
  while driving, 61–62
  faulty, 43
  in musculoskeletal pain, 154–56
Power of Positive Thinking, The (Peale), 106–7
Pregnancy, 81, 139
Prescription drugs, 87, 143
President's Committee on Employment of People with Disabilities, 35
Presleep routine, 84–86
Primary care physician, 44, 160–61, 168, 169
Professional counseling, 92
Proline, 137
Proteins, 129, 130, 136, 142
Prothrombin, 135
Prozac, 80–81

Quality of life, xii, 1–9
  gardening and, 24–25
  mind in, 106
  sleep and, 76

tools for improving, 170–74
travel and, 55

Radio-frequency energy, 78
Reaching overhead, 10
Reactive hypoglycemia, 58–59, 130–31
Reading in bed, 87–88
Relationships, 8, 91–105
  snoring and, 77
Relaxation exercises, 110
Repetitive motion disorder (RMD), 42
Repetitive motion injury (RMI), 42
Repetitive motions, 10
Repetitive strain injury (RSI), 40, 42–50
  warning signals of, 43–44
Research, 4
Research funding, 175–76
Resentment, 92, 93, 98–99
Rest
  with RSI, 46
Rest breaks
  while driving, 65
Restless leg syndrome, 87
Restless legs, 136
Restorative sleep, 76
  herbs as aid to, 81–82
  lack of, 6
Rheumatoid arthritis, 8, 110, 111, 175–76
Rheumatologist(s), 44, 161
Rhyme
  as memory aid, 123
Right brain/left brain, 117–18
Roles, 91, 125–26
Routines, 122
RSI
  see Repetitive strain injury (RSI)

Russell, I. Jon, and Jenny Fransen
   Fibromyalgia Help Book, The, 158

Sadness, 92
Seasonal affective disorder
   (SAD), 134
Self-image, 95
Self-respect, loss of, 10–11
Self-talk, 9, 86, 89, 165
Sense of control, 3, 110
Sense of humor, 123, 159
Serine, 137
Serotonin, 4–5, 139, 150
   deficiency in, 80, 81, 113–14
   and sleep, mood, pain percep-
      tion, 138
Sewing, 21–22
Sexual intimacy, 95–98
Sexuality
   healthy beliefs about, 95–96
Shoes, 69–72
   heels, 70–71
   insoles, 71
   shopping for, 72
   soles, 70, 71
   uppers, 71
Shopping for food, 20–21
Shoulder strain, 50
Showa Denko, 80
Side effects, xii, 46, 79, 121
   herbs, 82
Simplification, 6–8
Sit rather than stand, 17, 22
Sitting, 34
   in car, 61
   pain from, 58
   at work 40–42
Skullcap, 81
Sleep, xi, 8, 73–90
   away from home, 65, 66, 67
   and cognitive problems, 121

dysfunctional, 113
hours required, 83–84
lack of, 124
moving in, 89
preparations promoting, 78–82
slow wave, deep, 31
training body and mind for,
   86–87
tryptophan as aid to, 138
Sleep aids
   timing taking of, 85
Sleep apnea, 75
Sleep disrupters, 75–78
Sleep dysfunction, 73–75
Sleep hygiene, 28, 76, 82–86, 144,
   171
   basic rule of, 83
Sleep-phase syndrome disorder,
   76
Sleep problems, xii
   types of, 74
Sleep schedule, 30
   disruption of, 60
Sleep scientists, 74
Sleep specialists, 88
Sleep study, 75–76, 171
Sleepiness, 130
Sleeping pills, 79, 84
Slow cooker, 19
Smoking, 47
Social life, 27–28, 29, 93
Somnus Medical Technologies, 78
Sound-conditioning machine, 77
Snoring, 77–78
Specialists, 160, 168, 169
   RSI patients, 44
Specific serotonin reuptake inhib-
   itor (SSRI), 139
Spinal manipulation, 47
Spiritual life, 9
Splints, 46

Square Foot Gardening (Bartholomew), 25
Stairs, 23
climbing, 69
Standards
of cleanliness, 11
rethinking, 28
unrealistically high, 1
Standing, 68
pain in, 27–28
Standing up for yourself, 157–76
Stanford Sleep Disorders and Research Center, 78
Stationary bicycle, 65, 148–49
Stiffness
morning, 89
pain causing, 108
from sitting, 42
Strengthening, 151
Strengthening exercises, 146, 147
with RSI, 46
Stress, 34–35, 47, 137
avoiding/managing, 3, 117–18
causing bruxism, 76
cortisol and, 5
mood and, 110–19
pain causing, 108
triggers, 116
Stress reduction, 1
Stress-related issues (work), 36
Stretching, 65, 151
before exercise, 152
before moving in bed/getting
out of bed, 89, 90
Stretching exercises, 26, 43, 146,
147
RSI, 46
Substance P, 4–5, 109, 113,
149–50
Sugar, refined, 47, 59, 130, 142
Sugar intake, 31

Sugar substitutes, 59
Support groups, 2, 94, 160, 161
Support system, 159–60
Symptoms, xi
of dehydration, 58
RSI, 44
Symptoms (FM), 130
chemical imbalances exacerbate, 6
sleep and, 73, 74
yeast overgrowth and, 141–42

Take charge of your life, xii–xiii, 9
Tasks, breaking down, 123, 125
Teens
and cleaning, 12, 13
Temperature extremes, 137
Temperature sensitivity and re-
spiratory issues (work), 37
Temporomandibular joint, 76
Tender points, xi, 82, 99
Tendinitis, 42
Tension (muscles)
pain and, 108, 109
Textbook of Medicine (Cecil), 164
Thing that bothers you most cri-
terion, 14
Thoracic outlet syndrome, 43
Thoughts/thinking, 107
automatic, 112–13
and mood, 111
negative, 86, 87, 107, 110–11,
112
positive, 107
Threonine, 137
Time zone changes, 59–61
"To-do" lists, 125
Tools, gardening, 27
Toxic substances, 137
Traeger method, 156
Training heart rate, 151–52

Trauma, 137
see also Cumulative trauma
Travel, 55–72
    by car, 61–65
    time zone changes and jet lag,
        59–61
    what to pack, 56–57
Treadmill, 65
Treatment(s), xii
    obstructive sleep apnea, 75–76
    RSI, 46
Treatment (FM)
    cognitive behavioral therapy,
        110–12
Tryptophan, 4, 84, 137, 138–39,
    142
Tylenol, 80
Tyrosine, 137, 139

Ulcers, 165
Unpleasantness, avoiding, 17
U.S. Food and Drug Administra-
    tion (FDA), 78, 80
U.S. National Institutes of
    Health, 175

Valerian, 81
Valine, 137
Vasquez, Ernesto, 105
Vervain, 81
Visiting, 65–67
Vitamin A, 131–32, 134
Vitamin B$_3$ (niacin), 132
Vitamin B$_6$, 47, 138
Vitamin B$_{12}$, 131
Vitamin C, 47, 131, 132, 135
Vitamin D, 131–34, 135
Vitamin E, 47, 131–32

Vitamin K, 134–35
Vitamin supplements, 128,
    131–35
    guide to, 133–34t
    risk in, 143–44

Wakefulness, 74
Wakening too often/too early, 74,
    88–89
Walking, 65, 68–72, 146
    guidelines for, 152–53
    painful, 20, 63
Water, 58, 60, 66, 151
Water retention, 46
Water-soluble vitamins, 131, 132
Well-being, sense of
    in gardening, 25
Wellbutrin, 139
Wheeled transportation
    at airports, 57
White noise, 77
Women
    life roles, 92
Work, 11, 92
    accommodations at, 33–40
    strategies at, 33–54
    working out at, 52–54
Work surface, 41–42
Workers' compensation, 44
World Wide Web site, 143
Writing things down, 122

Yeast elimination diet, 130
Yeast overgrowth, 140–43

Zoloft, 139
Zolpidem tartrate (Ambien), 79,
    84